CAROLYN FAULDER is a journalist and writer, who specialises in social and health subjects (especially as they relate to women's lives), careers information and the promotion of better opportunities for women in all areas. She was a feature writer for *Nova* until 1975 and has contributed to a variety of publications, including the *Sunday Times*, the *Guardian*, *Good Housekeeping* and *Cosmopolitan*. She is co-author of *The Women's Directory* (Quartet 1976) and *Treat Yourself to Sex* (Penguin 1980). Her other books are *Talking to Your Doctor* (Virago 1978) and *Cosmopolitan's Career's Guide* (1979). She lives in London.

Carolyn Faulder's interest in breast cancer and the controversial issues its treatment raises for women arose out of work she did as a journalist in the early seventies. She is at present involved in two working parties, one concerned with the setting up of a clinical trial comparing different forms of treatment, the other monitoring the progress of the national breast cancer screening trial described in this book. She is strongly convinced that one of the ways to achieve better and more effective health care is to improve co-operation and understanding between doctors and patients, basing these efforts on mutual respect and an open sharing of knowledge. *Breast Cancer* is the authoritative work on the detection and treatment of one of the most intimidating health problems a woman has to face. Honest, positive and reassuring, it answers the many questions that cause patients and their families the greatest anxiety.

Carolyn Faulder

Breast Cancer

a guide to early detection and treatment

Published by VIRAGO PRESS Limited 1982
Ely House, 37 Dover Street, London W1X 4HS
First published by Pan Books Limited 1979
Copyright © Carolyn Faulder 1979, 1982
Printed and bound by J. W. Arrowsmith,
Winterstoke Road, Bristol

British Library Cataloguing in Publication Data
Faulder, Carolyn
    Breast cancer.—2nd ed.
    1. Breast—Cancer
    I. Title
    616.99'449   RC280.B8
    ISBN 0-086068-287-0

Contents

This book remembers with affection, admiration and gratitude two women whose lives and work have been a source of inspiration to me and many others:

Moira Keenan, former editor of *The Times* Women's Page, and a very dear friend who was ever warm-hearted, generous, brave and joyous

Caroline Nicholson, journalist, whose frank, informed articles on this subject in the early seventies broke down the barriers of taboo and fear

Introduction

This is a book about breast cancer. It contains hard facts, good facts, hopeful facts, sad facts, interesting facts, plain facts about the past treatment of this disease and present control of it, and, finally, some cautiously encouraging facts which give us reason to expect a much higher rate of cure and possibly prevention in the not so distant future. This is a book for people whose desire to know the truth outweighs their natural dread of a potentially but by no means always fatal disease. I have written it in the belief that to be armed with all the facts is the only sane way to confront the enemy, whenever and wherever it may appear – within me, you or your nearest and dearest.

There is one fact I do lack – the personal knowledge of what it feels like to be told: 'You have breast cancer.' Obviously, I hope I will not have this particular experience but I also hope that my lack of it will not disqualify me in the eyes of those readers who have, as therefore being someone who cannot possibly understand what it means to hear those words. Like many women over 35 I have had my frights, having twice found lumps which were then aspirated as cysts. Also, like most of us – men and women – I have friends who have had breast cancer and I have talked to many other women in the same situation, strangers introduced to me because they think it is essential that women should be informed as fully as possible about all aspects of breast cancer; *before* it happens, should that turn out to be their destiny. Several of these women regret their own lack of knowledge about the disease when the blow did hit them and a few feel that they were deliberately kept in the dark by the hospital staff – for reasons which will be discussed later in this book – but they hope that through sharing their experiences and difficulties with me, the women who read this book will be encouraged and strengthened rather than downcast. Certainly their courage, their optimism, their frankness and their determination to discover and accept the truth has been a tremendous source of inspiration to me.

To them and to the many doctors, researchers, nurses, social scientists, psychologists, and other experts who are dedicated to the cause of reducing the incidence rate and mortality rate of breast cancer, and to lessening the suffering it can cause – psychological often more than physical – I owe an enormous debt of gratitude. So many hours of so many busy people's time have been spared to me, explaining patiently and carefully to a partially ignorant laywoman, what their work involves, what they are trying to achieve, how they justify their method of treatment, which areas of research are ripe and promising for development and which others, such as the psychological care of mastectomy patients, have been sadly and badly neglected for too long. They too have been gratifyingly open with me, admitting their doubts and their failures – here I think particularly of the medical profession – as well as signalling to me areas of success and generously introducing me to colleagues whose work they believe to be valuable and should be known about more widely.

It would be invidious to mention names when all have been so helpful but I would like to record a special thank-you to the many members of the British Breast Group who welcomed me in their surgeries, offices and clinics round the country. As the name suggests, this is a small band of people united by their common long-standing dedication and their enthusiasm – shared by many others in this field, both in this country and all over the world. This united effort seems to me to offer women the best chance they have that this disease will finally be licked. They will certainly not agree with everything they read in this book, nor will they expect to, since they don't agree on everything among themselves. I hope, however, they will think that I have fairly represented their differing points of view. Particular mention must, however, be made of Dr Maureen Roberts and Betty Wolpert who read the book in manuscript. Their helpful comments and criticisms saved me from errors of fact and understanding.

Now it is my turn to be honest. I confess that I did not start this book with any great enthusiasm. Cancer is as frightening a

concept for me as it is for most other people and the prospect
of being immersed in research about a certain manifestation of
the disease to which my age and sex make me especially vulnerable filled me with quiet gloom rather than the pleasant antici-
pation I usually feel about a new book. However, as time went on
and I learnt more about the disease, some of it considerably more
disturbing than I had imagined, I nonetheless felt my own des-
pair lifting. At least I was beginning to understand what it was all
about, what it would mean to have breast cancer, what one could
hope for in terms of survival and quality of life. A lot of that
information is good and shows every sign of getting better fast,
but there is no place for false optimism.

Writing this book has been a personal voyage of discovery. I
have seen at first hand the remarkable persistence of an inquiring
scientific mind, been impressed by the marvellous resilience of the
human spirit, and, most important of all, I have learnt that while
knowledge does not necessarily kill fear, it can render it impotent.

'You have set yourself a difficult task,' said one woman cancer
specialist to me. 'It is that of giving information which must be
accurate, maintaining hope which is essential and avoiding fear
which is unnecessary.'

As a general indication of the contents, Parts One and Two
present an over-view of the whole subject of breast cancer, including current knowledge about the origins and behaviour of the
disease, methods of diagnosis and treatment and a consideration
of certain controversial subjects such as screening and the ethics
of controlled clinical trials. Part Three is devoted to the special
situation of the woman who has had a mastectomy and who
requires information and guidance to help her adjust to the
effects this operation may have on her life and her personal relationships. I have aimed to clarify medical names and phrases as
they first appear in the text, but both the subject and its termin-
ology are complex, so a glossary is included.

I hope that the readers who follow me through this book will
share my conviction that the journey of enlightenment is worthwhile. I think of them as my *alter ego* and I have not, therefore,
withheld any part of the truth about breast cancer which I would

not wish to know myself. That means recording all that I have
learnt about the disease and its treatment at this present moment
in history. My best hope for the future is that ten years from now
this book will be completely out of date.

Author's note: for explanations of terms used in this book, refer
to the index or the glossary.

part one

On guard

1 Bosom thoughts

Attitudes

It has become a fashionable cliché to say that we live in a breast obsessed society. Never before, it is constantly said, has so much attention, and money, been devoted to exposing this delicate and beautiful part of a woman's body. Breasts are exalted as the epitome of all that is most feminine and desirable in a woman. Their size, their shape, their uplift, their cleavage, their presentation, with and without covering, are the subject of endless discussions, articles and pictures. Breasts are exhibited to sell anything and everything from newspapers to night storage heaters, toffees to tractors. They are the basic stock-in-trade of the adman's art and the romantic novelist's passionate pen.

But nothing that we know or read about, or see in the visual arts of other periods and other cultures, can lead us to suppose that the female bosom was ever anything but very important. There has never been a time or a place when men have not been fascinated and enchanted by its curves. They have sought to reproduce its harmonious beauty in a variety of ways and for a variety of reasons – religious, sexual and artistic – not only by straightforward imitation but in the shape of their artefacts and even their weapons. Pots, vases, bowls, shields and helmets all mirror the female breast, and there are many other man-made objects, ancient and modern, some created for worship, others for aesthetic pleasure, which produce the same sensuous impression; at least as many as those which reflect the phallic image.

The child begins its life at its mother's breast and never entirely loses its need for the warmth, comfort, nourishment and sensual delight that it offers. If the child grows into a woman she enjoys the pleasure of offering her own breasts to her lover and to her child, but a boy grown into a man must find other women to replace the first woman in his life. Occasionally a man is so jealous of his wife's breasts that he refuses to allow her to breastfeed their child for fear that this will ruin their shape. Not true, incidentally, providing that she cares for them during and after pregnancy by wearing a bra of the proper size and support, and rubs oil into them to prevent stretch marks and cracked nipples.

A woman's attitude to her breasts is influenced by the society she lives in, as much as by the physical facts of her own make-up and the personal tastes of the men she encounters. No one could deny that the female bosom is exploited in our twentieth-century culture, but has there ever been a time or a civilization when it was not? Indeed, there may well have been periods when the exposure was much more blatant and provocative.

Fashion tells us a good deal more about the way people actually lived and thought than any historian's theory and, looking at the records earlier civilizations have left us, there seem to be few periods when the bosom was not, quite literally, prominent. James Laver, the fashion historian, suggests, in his uniquely witty and plausible way, that the clothes we wear unconsciously reflect our relationship to the opposite sex. Most of human history has been dominated by patriarchal societies so men have dressed on the class-conscious 'hierarchical principle' - on the whole formally and pompously - to impress women with their status and capacity to provide. Women, on the other hand, having to rely almost entirely on their looks and powers of attraction to win a man, a home, security and minimum respect, have dressed alluringly, embodying the sex-conscious 'seduction principle'. Calculated exposure is the basic feature of this principle, but since men are easily bored, the focus has constantly altered. Bosoms, legs, ankles, feet, wrists, necks, waists, indeed every tiny portion of the female anatomy has been the object of male lustful interest at one time or another, constituting what the psychologist J. C. Flugel calls 'the shifting erogenous zone'.

Bosoms, however, have been more constantly erogenous than most. Even at periods when religious taboos have been at their height, men and women have found ways of evading moral disapproval, like the Renaissance painters who would use their beautiful mistresses as a model for the Virgin Mother tenderly offering her perfect breast to the Holy Infant.

Laver also points out that during the periods when women have achieved a measure of emancipation, their clothes correspondingly reflect an indifference to male approval. Instead they dress to please themselves, which may be either comfortably or 'shamelessly'. He believes that that process of change towards emancipation is now irreversible, hence the dominance of the 'utility principle' where, neither sex having a need to impress the other, dress becomes androgynous. His theory could explain another characteristic of our modern Western society which finds expression in the crudely commercial exploitation of women's bodies, and particularly their breasts, sometimes to the point of freakishness. Could this be man's way of exacting his revenge for woman's escape from his control? Or maybe it is because men have never outgrown their childish awe of the big-bosomed earth mother, nor perhaps found new sexual outlets to compensate for their sense of loss which makes so many of them project their unsubtle fantasies into every facet of our day-to-day lives. Whatever the reason, the fact is that, pleasurably or not, we are obliged to swallow big boobs with our morning juice, see them bending over us in gross outline from the hoardings as we travel to and from work and find it impossible to avoid their thrusting presence as we read our newspapers, flick through magazines, look at a film or watch television.

Women may complain at the way men make capital out of their bodies but are they so blameless themselves? Exploitation will certainly never cease until women themselves stop conniving at it. Just by thinking in the male terms of 'under-privileged' and 'well-endowed' a woman is denying scientific evidence and her own experience which tell her that size and shape have little to do with sexual gratification and are most unlikely to affect her ability to breastfeed, should she want to. Yet what woman has not lamented and agonized at some time in her life about her breasts, either because she thinks they are too big or too small, not round enough or too saggy, or because they appeared too early or too late. A woman rightly feels that her breasts express something of her essential femininity and the man who loves her will support her in that belief, but always remember that they are only a part, never the whole, of what makes her a woman.

Facts

The human breast is a paired mammary gland which first appears as a minute swelling in the six-week-old foetus. By the time the child is born, boy and girl alike, it will have an elementary internal system of large milk ducts and, externally, two nipples each surrounded by a small circle of deeper pink which is called the areola. The breasts remain flat in both sexes until puberty. For a girl this is usually between the ages of 11 and 13 when she starts secreting the hormones oestrogen and progesterone. These cause many changes in her body, but the most obvious external one is her developing bosom. The areola swells slightly while internally ducts begin to grow inwardly, branching out into smaller ducts which end in tiny milk-producing glands. Each of these ducts is contained in lobular segments of tissue which are embedded in fat and separated from each other by fibrous tissue. The ducts converge like the spokes of a wheel on to a central reservoir just behind the areola where the milk collects when a woman is lactating (secreting milk) after childbirth. There may be anything from twelve to twenty lobules in the breast and each has its own fine opening through the nipple. As the adolescent girl grows into a fully adult woman these lobular structures develop further and more fat accumulates which gives the young female breast its characteristically round firm shape. The size of the breast depends on the amount of fatty and fibrous tissue there is, and not on the glandular element which is concentrated in the central and upper part.

The breast tissue is attached to the underlying pectoral (chest) muscles and the overlying skin by fine ligaments. If any of these strands which are called Cooper's ligaments become cancerous, they contract, causing the breast to dimple or become fixed to the chest wall. The breast is basically hemispherical in shape but it does have a tongue-like extension leading into the armpit which is called the tail of the breast or the axillary tail. Axilla is the medical term for armpit and is worth remembering because it occurs frequently in this book to describe the position of certain very important lymph nodes. The lymph nodes are small masses of gland tissues all over the body through which lymph, a colourless fluid, similar to blood but without the red corpuscles, drains and is purified. They are a vital part of the body's defence mechanism against disease and they are discussed in greater detail in Chapters 7, 8 and 10. In the breast area, there are, in addition to the axillary nodes, the pectoral nodes which run behind the breast and up the outer side, the subclavicular nodes just below the collar bone, the supraclavicular nodes just above the inner half of the collar bone, and the internal mammary nodes which run in a chain between the two breasts.

Unfortunately, breasts give trouble as well as pleasure. Subject to endless hormonal assaults from puberty onwards, they are frequently sore, sometimes extremely painful for years on end without relief. Pain does not mean cancer. Indeed, quite the contrary as cancer usually makes it first appearance in the breast without this warning but you should always consult a doctor if you have persistent pain.

This book is about understanding and coping with the darker side of having breasts which threatens any woman of any age.

2 A royal curse

Leave her to heaven,
And to those thorns that in her bosom lodge,
To prick and sting.

So cries the tormented ghost of Hamlet's father after revealing to his outraged son the crimes which have been committed by his faithless wife and rapacious brother. He specifically begs Hamlet not to harm his mother physically as he believes that in time her conscience will torture her enough, but in Shakespeare's mind the imagery of thorns and hurt could have come from an actual experience of seeing a relative or neighbour die of breast cancer. It also suggests the primitive fear that there is no final escape from our wrongdoing.

'Why me? What have I done to deserve this?' is a question that many cancer patients ask themselves. Obviously, no one ever deserves cancer, but the reasons why breast cancer picks out one woman and not another when both may seem, to a medical eye, evenly matched in most respects, remain inscrutable. Apart from excessive radiation there are no environmental links, as with cigarettes for lung cancer, and other possible agents, to be discussed in this chapter, are still no more than suspicions; some, however, show growing signs of being well founded.

Cancer has always been a disease of mankind and traces of it have been found in very ancient human remains, but since it is primarily a disease of old age, proportionately fewer of the total population would have been afflicted by it. Such evidence as we have about methods of treatment sound crude and unavailing for the most part; in the case of breast cancer, there are indications that tumours were being cut out with knives as early as 1500 BC. However, by the first century AD, Celsus, a Roman writer, was advising against the more radical surgery which involves removing the chest wall muscles behind the breast tissue.

This was progressive thinking then and, in the eyes of those surgeons who still favour the Halsted operation, as it is now called, (see Chapter 8) would be considered no less advanced today. It is both staggering and dismaying to realize that surgical amputation has been the norm, indeed the only treatment for breast cancer for thousands of years. Anaesthetic and antiseptics were introduced little more than a hundred years ago, so it is no wonder that many women like Attossa, the wife of the Greek King, and Madame Poisson, the mother of Madame de Maintenon, preferred to endure the tumour, however terrible, than the barbarism of the surgeon's knife. And it is only very recently, within the last five to ten years, that treatment other than surgery, and to a lesser degree radiotherapy, is being considered as a serious adjunct, if not an alternative, to amputation, for many more cases than those once deemed 'inoperable'.

It tends to be those doctors with the greatest experience of breast cancer who are the most willing to admit that even now their ignorance is probably greater than their knowledge. This is because so many basic questions still await answers. Apart from not knowing what causes breast cancer, no one has yet established whether there are several types of disease; whether it is multi-factorial in origin (more than one cause); whether, if left long enough, it invariably metastasizes (spreads into other parts of the body and develops secondary tumours). Diagnostic techniques are still not refined enough always to make a definite distinction between an 'early' or a 'late' tumour, and prognostic indices for the patient's future can be equally unreliable.

A few figures

The field of breast cancer studies is mined with suspicions but so far there has been no explosion of certainty about anything except, unfortunately, the mortality figures. For women aged between 35 to 54, it is the leading cause of death. In Britain one woman in seventeen will develop the disease and one woman in thirty can eventually expect to die of it. In 1977, the last year for which there are recorded figures, 11,820 women died of breast cancer. There are indications that the disease is changing biologically. Not only do some doctors think that it may be getting more malignant, it is striking more young women and women generally. In Great Britain alone it has been increasing at the rate of more than 1 per cent per year for the last twenty years.

After this litany of woe, you may well wonder whether it is worth reading any further, since if so little is known can anything be done to improve the chances of cure? The answer is surprising and optimistic, mainly because of some very concentrated re-thinking and research which has been going on among small groups of people, all over the world, who are determined to devote the same energy to tackling breast cancer as has recently been devoted to leukaemia in children, and Hodgkin's disease, with very good results.

I deliberately trotted out the black statistics first so that they could be absorbed and then put behind you. However, one thing worth remembering in connection with the mortality rate is that although breast cancer is particularly lethal in the middle years, it is by no means the chief cause of death in women as a whole. Only 4 per cent of women die each year in this country from breast cancer, compared with 14 per cent from respiratory diseases, 17 per cent from strokes and 22 per cent from coronary disease. (Minister of State for Health, quoted in Hansard, November 1974.)

Incidentally, men can get breast cancer too. One in every 100 cases is male; he is usually elderly and certainly never younger than 40. The tumour is usually central, close to the nipple and treatment is along the same lines as for women.

The next important point to grasp is that there is a very thin line between knowing for sure, and producing tightly argued theories based on well-grounded hypotheses for pursuing certain courses of action. In the scientific world nothing can be proved positive until every possible negative has been ruled out but that does not prevent clever people following a hunch and making sure that their tracks are well observed, in the event of success, by setting up strictly controlled clinical trials. This is what is happening with dramatic effect in every area of breast cancer studies and the fact that the more that is discovered the more complicated does the disease reveal itself to be, is encouraging in one respect. It gives doctors a greater challenge and more scope for action, and it is in their nature and their training to want to be doing. Otherwise, we, and they, may begin to question their function and whether they are really helping their patients.

Epidemiology is the name given to the scientific study of the distribution and determinants of disease in the community. As in most other disciplines, epidemiologists tend to specialize in a particular disease – epidemics originally, as the name suggests – but since most of those have now been brought under control their area of interest has widened and so also have their terms of reference. Their main aim is to find clues about the causes (aetiology) of a particular disease and in doing so they look at several significant factors such as the distribution of the disease – in what parts of the world it is most prevalent and among what populations; whether it is age or sex linked; whether there seem to be certain 'high-risk' factors and 'high-risk' groups of people; whether it appears to be genetic, environmental, viral or degenerative in origin, or possibly a combination of some or all of these things. The epidemiologist must combine the most exacting eye for detailed analysis with inexhaustible thoroughness as he sifts through the evidence, together with an instinctive 'nose' for clues.

Clues to causes

In breast cancer there are now several important clues which are being followed up. Among the most significant are those relating to a woman's reproductive history, which indicate that hormones undoubtedly play a part. Favourable factors are having a baby before you are twenty (less than one half the risk of the general population); having a late menarche (first menstruation); having an early menopause (before the age of 45) or having an artificial menopause by having your ovaries removed between the age of 35 and 45. (This is done by surgery or radiation and is called an oopherectomy.) It used to be thought that having lots of babies and breastfeeding them were also protective factors but later studies have shown these to be of no significance either way.

The corresponding 'high-risk' factors are having your menarche early, before the age of 13; having a late menopause after the age of 50; and having your first baby after the age of 35 or not having children at all (nulliparous). As long ago as 1713, an Italian physician, Ramazzini, observed that nuns seemed to be more prone to breast cancer than their married sisters. (Conversely, they seldom, if ever, get cancer of the cervix which is now known to bear a close relation to the number of sexual partners a woman has and the age at which she starts sexual intercourse.)

Other factors which must be taken into account when assessing a woman's vulnerability to breast cancer are where she lives and what is her race. North American and West European women are the most prone, whereas if you are an Asian or a black African the likelihood is reduced dramatically. Furthermore, the disease in these countries appears to be less aggressive. An interesting fact which epidemiologists love to quote but which puzzles them enormously is that although Japanese women living in Japan are the least likely of all populations to get breast cancer, their risk increases as soon as they emigrate to North America and becomes progressively worse with each successive generation. The change to a high-fat diet has been suggested and diet has also been blamed for the generally increasing rate of breast cancer in all the Western countries with similar eating habits, but to date no definite facts have been produced to support this view.

A woman's age is very important. Before the age of 30 she is very unlikely to get breast cancer, even if she has a long history of producing lumps and bumps (which, incidentally, she should always take to her doctor). As she moves into her late thirties and even more so into her forties, approaching the menopause, her risk climbs steeply, levelling out to some extent after the age of 50 which is one factor suggesting that there is a biological difference in the disease between pre-menopausal and post-menopausal women. Women in their sixties and seventies again become increasingly vulnerable.

The possibility that breast cancer can be inherited is now under close investigation, since it is a fact that women whose mothers or sisters, or other close relatives on the maternal side have had breast cancer run a doubled risk themselves. This suggests that they may inherit not the disease itself but a genetic predisposition to it, arising perhaps from hormonal make-up acting in conjunction with certain other factors. This risk goes up even more for a woman whose mother had the disease before her menopause, or had it in both breasts.

Could the disease be caused by a virus? is another question epidemiologists are asking. For a while it was thought that it could be transmitted through breastmilk but this now appears to have been ruled out.

A further group of women who are more prone to breast cancer are those who have previously had cancer in one breast or in some other parts of the body. Also it appears that as women get older, those who suffer a certain type of benign breast disease called variously fibrocystic disease or chronic cystic mastitis run an extra risk. In medical terms, a benign disease is one producing growths or a tumour which may mimic cancer symptoms but are not malignant.

At our present state of knowledge it is quite impossible to categorize these risks in order of importance, especially as they are likely to work in combination rather than singly, but everything points the strongest finger of suspicion at hormones. So far we have only discussed the possible effect of endogenous hormones (those which are produced internally by the ovaries and certain glands) but if they are as relevant as the evidence suggests, then it follows that we should also be considering the effect of exogenous hormones (those which are administered externally). This means that the Pill, the oestrogens given in hormone replacement therapy (HRT) and hormones administered for other reasons such as averting a miscarriage, preventing lactation or preventing conception (the 'morning after' pill) should all be looked at much more closely for any possible link with breast cancer. Oestrogen probably does not cause cancer but it could create a receptive environment for it, under certain conditions.

What about the Pill?

For quite a while it was considered that the Pill had a positively protective effect against breast cancer, a view based mainly on studies showing that women who use the Pill for two or more years appear less likely to get benign breast disease; further investigation suggests that it is the progesterone rather than the oestrogen in the Pill which causes this.

There are currently three major studies in the United Kingdom surveying large groups of women on the Pill to see whether there is any link between the Pill and breast cancer, and there are similar ones in the United States, started rather later. Preliminary findings coming from the one run by the Royal College of General Practitioners (unpublished at the date of writing) suggest that there could be a small increase in risk for young women who take the Pill for a long time. Because of the emotional overtones attached to any observations about the Pill, and the many 'ifs' and 'buts' hedging research into it, the scientists hesitate to commit themselves until they are reasonably certain, for fear of causing a wave of panic. Nonetheless women should know about these reservations when weighing up the pros and cons of oral contraception.

According to Professor Martin Vessey, an epidemiologist with a special interest in exogenous hormones, who is running the other two studies from an Oxford base, 'the Pill is going to be an enigma with regard to cancer for another ten years at least' and he gives three very cogent reasons why this should be so.

First, there is the fact of the changing pattern of use. When the Pill was first introduced into this country in the early sixties its main takers were married women in their thirties who had completed their families and wanted to avoid any 'mistakes'. Now the situation has quite reversed, reinforced by the recently published contra-indications for the Pill being taken by women over 35, especially if they are also heavy smokers. Oral contraceptives are now extensively used by young women in their teens and early twenties to prevent a first pregnancy. One of Professor Vessey's on-going investigations is a case-control study in which he has interviewed 707 women who contracted breast cancer before the age of 50. This is a remarkably large study of its kind, yet out of that number only twenty women were on the Pill before their first pregnancy. If a similar study were to be launched ten years from now, he is certain that the vast majority would be in that position, perhaps producing vastly different conclusions.

The second important fact is that as yet there are no satisfactory figures about long-term users, for the simple reason that there are very few women who have been consistently on the Pill since it was first available. Again Professor Vessey's study reveals that only eighteen women in it have been taking the Pill for longer than eight years and many of these have not done so continuously. As it is well known that carcinogenic agents are often latent for twenty to thirty years it is essential for the epidemiologists to scrutinize a whole generation of long-term users before they can come to definite conclusions.

Finally, there is the fact of the changed nature of the Pill itself. Certain types of pill are no longer in use and new varieties are constantly being introduced, tending all the time to lower dosages of the oestrogen component.

These three important considerations combined with the belief that breast cancer is almost certainly multifactorial in origin present an amazingly complicated pre-menopausal pattern of possibilities for the researchers to unravel.

The picture is almost as baffling when looking at women on the far side of 50, mainly because so little has been done in the way of sustained investigation into the relationship between HRT and breast cancer. In the United States where many more women for very much longer have been taking oestrogen for menopausal symptoms, and afterwards, in pursuit of the Feminine Forever dream, a causal connection has been established for endometrial cancer (lining of the uterus) but so far nothing clearcut has emerged about breast cancer. It does, however, appear that women who use these oestrogens for more than four years run a significantly greater risk of developing benign breast disease.

With so many studies going on and new evidence constantly being turned up it is obvious that we still have some time to wait before we can be sure of what we are doing to our bodies when we take that daily pill. Meanwhile what are we to think, and more importantly what should we do? Professor Vessey probably echoes the necessarily cautious thinking of his fellow researchers when he commits himself this far: 'I find it hard to believe that the Pill has no effect on the disease. It seems biologically highly improbable. The possibility of a hazardous effect in women otherwise at high-risk is particularly worth watching.'

Other possibilities

Excessive doses of radiation have been briefly mentioned as causes inducing breast cancer. Evidence for this is incontrovertible from three different sources. First, there is the aftermath of Hiroshima where an excessive number of Japanese women (especially ironic in view of their normally low vulnerability) developed breast cancer, most of them being between the ages of 14 and 19 when the bomb was dropped. The other two groups of women known to be victims of radiation are those who were exposed to large doses of X-rays during the course of treatment for tuberculosis or for chronic mastitis in the days when the potential harmfulness of such treatment was still not recognized.

From earliest times, people have speculated as to whether cancer could be activated by psychological factors. Galen, a Greek physician, divided women into melancholic and sanguine types. The former who suffered from 'an excess of bile' were the ones likely to develop breast cancer. He also, much more pertinently, observed that regular menstruation kept women healthy and that most breast tumours developed after the menopause. There have been many studies attempting to show a relationship between stress, or a severe loss – such as the death of a spouse, child or other beloved person – and cancer. Scientists are hesitant to accept them as more than interesting speculations because, by their nature, they are difficult to prove.

However, that there may be some relationship between personality and a predisposition to certain illnesses has gained more credibility recently, especially since Professor Friedman defined a

'Type A' personality – intensely ambitious, restless and driving with a tendency to choose careers dominated by deadlines – which was more likely to suffer from heart attacks. Now some research carried out at King's College Hospital suggests that there could also be a 'Type C' for cancer. Between 1973 and 1974 a total of 160 women who were admitted for biopsy because of a lump in their breast were put through exhaustive personality and life history questionnaires, the answers to which were then checked out with husbands or close relatives. Of these women, sixty-nine turned out to have breast cancer and the remainder had benign disease. Stress, depression, an introverted rather than extroverted personality – all factors which have been suspected in connection with cancer – appeared to be unimportant, but women with 'an abnormal release of emotions' were much more frequent in the breast cancer group. Mainly these were people who tended to bottle up their feelings. Most said that they could only remember losing their temper once or twice in their lives and some were positive that they had never done so. A smaller group of women, also with breast cancer, admitted to losing their temper at least once a month and generally being much more emotional. The women with benign disease appeared more moderate, 'apparently normal' as the researchers are careful to define it, in the expression of their emotions.

One hesitates to make too much of such findings particularly as they are based on a very small sample, for fear that people will automatically classify themselves as 'high risks'. They certainly don't suggest that personality *causes* cancer, but it is just possible that it could be an added risk factor when it is combined with certain physical risks.

Having run through the known possible factors which may cause breast cancer and, who knows, the vital mystery factor X may yet remain to be discovered, this is probably the moment to clear up a few misconceptions which can cause women needless worry and unhappiness. A knock, a blow or a fall does *not* cause breast cancer. It is not infectious and it is not, strictly speaking, hereditary, except in the rather remote sense that a daughter may, but does not necessarily, inherit her mother's constitutional characteristics.

However, a definite profile does emerge of certain groups of women who can be defined as 'high risk'. The next chapter looks at what is available and what we should be hoping for, to help such women in particular, as well as women generally, to safeguard themselves against breast cancer.

3 What are we looking for?

There are only two ways in which we are going to improve the cure rates for breast cancer. The first is by earlier detection (diagnosis) and the second is by finding better methods of treatment. Nobody disputes these two essential points but among the experts there is plenty of argument and disagreement, about which is the more important and, therefore, deserves more resources devoted to it and, within the two areas, which are the best methods to use. The reason for the debate is quite simple. Nobody yet knows, for sure, that any one method works better than another; nobody has yet been able to prove, beyond doubt, that their preferred course of action produces positive and lasting results. There is no shortage of ideas and theories, but trying them out on an approved clinical trial basis takes time, money and a heavy concentration of skilled personnel, all of which are limited commodities especially when measured against other pressing areas of need within our National Health Service. Meanwhile, in the midst of so much uncertainty, women continue to get breast cancer and it is everyone's major concern to save their lives. This chapter looks at the simplest and easiest diagnostic aid which is available to every woman now, providing she will learn how to use it.

Breast self-examination

The supreme advantage of breast self-examination is that it enables a woman to familiarize herself with the shape, feeling and appearance of her breasts in a normal condition. In a more subtle way, it helps her to overcome any lingering inhibitions she may have about her body generally, so that should she find it necessary to visit her doctor because she thinks there may be something wrong with any part of her she will feel less reluctant about communicating her problem. (As we will see later on in this book, proper communication between doctor and patient is vital for diagnosis and treatment.) And it costs nothing except a little time – five minutes a month – and a certain amount of patience and, even more important, determination to learn to do it properly.

Most young girls are keenly interested in the development of their breasts and may spend long hours gazing at themselves in the mirror, usually agonizing quite unnecessarily because they don't measure up to some impossible ideal, which makes it all the more curious that so many older women seem almost afraid to look at their breasts, let alone touch them. If this is a problem for you, don't be ashamed of it. We are not all made the same, psychologically any more than physically, and some people are naturally more modest about their bodies or may find it more difficult to deny the effects of an upbringing which, by today's standards, may have been rather strict and prudish. For the sake of your own health, however, it is very important to overcome these inhibitions and the instructions on breast self-examination include suggestions for ways of breaking yourself in gently to the idea.

There is another very powerful reason why many women are turned off the idea of breast self-examination and it is one which doctors are acutely aware of but don't know how to combat. It is also very understandable. Women are frightened of what they may find. It isn't that they don't know that they should report anything unusual like a lump or a discharge; on the contrary, they think they know only too well what the doctor's verdict will be. Breast lumps are automatically associated with breast cancer and in the mind of a woman that so often means only two things: losing her breast and possibly her life. Yet it is a scientific fact that *only one in ten lumps* turns out to be cancer and if you are under 30, the probability that it is harmless is even higher. All the same, any abnormality should be reported, if only to put your mind at rest.

Many women have naturally lumpy breasts. Others suffer from benign disease of one sort or another which may fluctuate with the menstrual cycle, making the breasts swollen and painful at certain times in the month, usually just before the period.

Breasts also change internally as the woman grows older. From being dense, glandular structures admirably suited for their prime function of giving milk to a baby they gradually become less glandular and more fatty, until in a woman's later years, after the menopause, fat has almost entirely replaced the glandular portion, but this too eventually reduces, giving them a character- istically shrunken (atrophic) appearance in old age.

The woman who has trained herself to feel her breasts regularly and knows about these normal changes will not be alarmed by them and yet, just because she knows her breasts so well, she will also know how to pick up an unexpected change. This is yet another very important advantage of breast self-examination. The woman who knows her own breasts well can help the doctor who is making a clinical examination. One very experienced sur- geon who examines on average two thousand breasts a year, told me that he still sometimes finds himself searching for a lump but if the woman is trained in breast self-examination she will point it out to him because she lives with her breasts and knows where there is a slight but detectable difference.

This is all very well, you may be saying, but does it make any difference in the long run? Many women fear that by the time they find a lump it will be too late anyway and they use this as an excuse not to visit their doctor until they become even more alarmed, either because it is getting bigger or becoming painful. Certainly it would be more satisfactory to detect alterations in breast tissue (lesions) before they got to the lump stage and it can, as we shall see, sometimes be done with the use of certain mach- inery, but this is not yet a practical possibility for all women. Until it is, women are well advised to use the best diagnostic aids they have, their own eyes and hands because, whatever the trouble, slight or serious, it is *always* better to have it treated immediately.

Although ninety per cent of breast cancers present as a lump there are other warning signs which women should be on the look-out for when they do their monthly examination. Maybe you think you know them off by heart but just in case you forget or miss one out, why not copy out this list and slip it into the corner of the mirror when you do your examination?

Breast Change in shape
Change in size (usually larger but sometimes appears to be shrinking and feels harder)
Puckering or dimpling of the skin
Enlarged veins
Lump or thickening anywhere

Nipple Discharge (any colour, any consistency)
Retraction or drawing in
Rash on nipple or areola (brown skin surrounding the nipple)
Lump or thickening
Change in skin texture

Arm Swelling of upper arm
Swelling in the armpit or above the breast (enlarged lymph or pectoral nodes)

There are many illustrated leaflets available which give you a step-by-step guide to breast self-examination and the addresses of the organizations supplying them are listed on page 143. A couple of good films illustrating the technique have also been made, but you do need to see them at least twice if not more often before you can memorize them accurately. If you are a member of a women's organization, a trade union, or work for a company which offers a good health-care scheme to its employees, then it would be worth suggesting that one be hired and shown at a time when the maximum number of women can attend (addresses on page 143).

In my experience, and in the view of most doctors and health educators who are particularly interested in promoting breast self-examination, the best way of learning how to do it is by one-to-one example. Ideally, this should be a woman doctor, nurse or even a lay person who has been specially trained because she can then stand in front of the woman – she doesn't have to undress! – and show her how to feel her breasts exactly as one hopes she feels her own. Alfreda Marter, who is Director of the Oxford Cancer Information Association, with long experience in the field of cancer education, advising the medical profession as well as the general public, says that it took her years of lecturing before she hit on this simple truth. She tried films, illustrated slides and anything else that seemed appropriate but she realized that nothing quite made the impact she wanted until one day she decided to make it just that more personal.

'I went through the whole routine and then, when I had got them really interested, I took off my jacket and showed them exactly what to do, over my blouse. I'd got them relaxed by now,' and after that it was easy to tell them how they should imagine themselves sitting in front of the mirror at home, stripped to the waist and having a good look at themselves. 'In the end they're laughing because they're thinking how lopsided they look, or odd, and I can reassure them that if we all did a topless then and there we would find that we are all in the same boat – different shapes, different sizes.'

Mrs Marter is a gifted teacher but she is convinced that many more people could follow her example and that, if they did, breast self-examination would have a much better chance of being accepted as part of a woman's normal health and beauty routine, like cleaning your face of make-up or doing daily exercises.

Breast self-examination is neither difficult nor complicated once you have mastered the order of the actions, but in order to be of any use it does require the following three Rs from you: Regularity, Relaxation and Repetition. *Regularity* means choosing a day of the month and always doing it on that day, no matter what may have got crowded into it. Pre-menopausal women are advised to do it immediately after their period ends when their breasts are likely to be at their softest and least lumpy: women after the menopause should pick any day of the month, say the first, so long as they don't forget it.

Relaxation means giving yourself the peace and privacy that you need to carry out this examination in a concentrated, careful and unhurried way. For those women who may find it a strange procedure at first – and it does take getting used to – doing it in the bath is a nice way to start. You have to touch your body anyway, if you wash yourself properly, but drop the flannel and run your soapy hands over your breasts. This is a good way of feeling for lumps and it will make you feel much less nervous next time. You don't want to be interrupted in the middle of your examination because you might leave out a stage, so if there are people in the house who could disturb you, lock the door. It is only for five minutes! *Repetition* means doing exactly the same routine in the same order every time. Here it is:

Looking (Investigating)

1 Strip to the waist. Sit or stand in front of a mirror with a good light, your arms hanging comfortably by your sides and look at your breasts carefully, noting their shape, their size and whether they differ in any way from each other. One may be larger than the other or set higher. Get used to the way your breasts look, and how your nipples are placed and then remember that image, looking at yourself the same way next time and every time thereafter so that you can be sure of spotting a change should one occur.

2 Raise your arms above your head and, turning slightly from side to side, continue to gaze at your reflection very carefully, looking for any distortion or change in the outline of your breasts. Then look downwards at your nipples, checking for any unusual change in their position or appearance.

3 Place your hands on your hips and press firmly downwards and inwards until you feel your chest muscles tighten. Look for any unusual skin puckering or nipple retraction.

Feeling (Palpation)

1 Lie on your bed. Place a folded towel under your left shoulder and let your left arm lie by your side. Examine your left breast first with your right hand.
Placing the pads of your fingers first above your nipple, press firmly but gently round your breast – outwards, downwards, inwards, inwards and upwards. Continue this circular motion

spirally until you have covered the whole surface of your breast – at least two circles, possibly three depending on the size of your breast.

2 Raise your left arm and place your hand behind your head so that your arm is bent.
Repeat exactly the same spiral circular motion as described above.

3 Keeping your arm above your head apply the same gentle pressure with your fingertips to your whole armpit area.

Your left breast has now been thoroughly examined. Put the folded towel under your right shoulder and repeat exactly the same procedure for feeling your right breast.

Once you have done this two or three times you will really wonder why you ever worried about it. There is absolutely no need to do it more than once a month and, indeed, when you have finished your examination, providing you have found no change, you can forget about your breasts until the same day next month. But what if you do find something unusual? You must, without any delay at all, make an appointment to see your doctor. Do not, in the interval, press the lump or squeeze the nipple. Whatever it is, leave it alone.

4 I've got a lump in my breast

Seeing the doctor

About 95 per cent of breast lumps are found by the woman herself, or by her husband or lover but, as we saw in the previous chapter, these are not the only suspicious signs to look out for. Always remember that you are your own best judge of whether your breasts are in a healthy condition, just because you are so aware of them and they are such a sensitive, important part of your body. Therefore, anything slightly unusual in the appearance of your breasts must be reported immediately to your GP. Don't be afraid of what he may say or that he may laugh at you for being foolishly over-anxious about yourself.

Most family doctors are sensible, sympathetic people who take their patients' worries seriously, but don't imagine that they are gifted with telepathic powers. If you don't explain what is wrong with you the doctor is not going to be able to guess unless he happens to be an exceptionally sensitive person who can pick up anxiety vibrations from across the desk. Fortunately, some doctors do realize that they have a duty to help their patients through psychological problems as well as physical ones and they know how to listen for the things unsaid as well as look at the presenting symptoms.

Many women who are worried about their health find it very difficult, once they are actually in the doctor's surgery, to admit their anxiety. If the doctor is a man, and most GPs are – hence the practice of referring to them as 'he' – they may feel embarrassed to explain intimate problems, so they may use their child's health as an excuse for coming, or produce some very minor symptom like a sore throat or a vague pain in some other part of the body. The best doctors – the ones who believe that prevention is better than cure – are aware of these avoidance tactics and will make it a routine part of their practice to inquire about their patient's health in general. If they haven't seen her for some time they will find out whether she has had her annual cervical smear test, whether she has any unusual pain or discharge in her genital area and also suggest a breast examination. This is ideal medical practice but don't rely on getting it from your doctor. In the final analysis, you are responsible for your health so if you are concerned about something, don't hesitate to go to the doctor and explain, in as exact a way as you can, what it is.

Just as there are a few doctors who will do everything they can to help their patients out, there is a minority which is either too apathetic, too 'busy' or just too downright intolerant of patients to pay proper attention to them unless they are almost dead on their feet. There are also a few men doctors who are always going to be somewhat defensive or aloof towards their women patients, perhaps because they don't like women very much or because they are afraid that they're going to be accused of improper behaviour. This is obviously a rare attitude, particularly nowadays in large group practices where there is usually a nurse in attendance, but it is worth remembering that doctors have their private hang-ups as much as the rest of us.

The doctor to beware of is the one who looks at your lump, or whatever else it may be, somewhat perfunctorily, and then says, 'Nothing to worry about! Come back in a month if it's still there.' Even though it may mean an unpleasant few minutes, refuse to accept this for an answer and *never* wait to see what happens. Although it is hard to disagree with a doctor since you are in the vulnerable position of having consulted him because of his superior expertise, you can be certain that this is never a satisfactory answer. One breast specialist takes the view that if a woman is worried about the possibility of breast cancer, even without any symptoms, then that is a medical symptom in itself and justifies the GP referring her to a fully equipped breast unit where she can have a complete examination.

What's stopping you?

However, it would be most unfair always to blame doctors for delay in dealing with breast symptoms. We have seen that there are women who manage to get themselves as far as the surgery, but once actually sitting in front of the doctor, find it very difficult to open their mouths. Unfortunately, many of them belong to the same group of women, about 25 per cent, who on finding a lump, delay making that first important visit for three months or even longer, possibly more than a year. Why do they do this? Research shows that these days it is very unlikely to be due to ignorance. Rather it is fear which paralyses them; fear, first of all, that it will prove to be a cancer, and secondly, that they will lose a breast. But all women naturally share these fears, so what is the extra factor which makes one in four women delay so long? It seems that age, class, education, marital status, pain, or absence of it, and many other indicators which psychologists use for measurement purposes have little or no bearing on women's behaviour in this situation, but they do share one common personality characteristic; they tend, in all the stressful conditions they meet in life, to deny their gravity, or even go so far as to pretend that they are not really happening. Thus when they feel a lump, they will immediately reassure themselves: 'it can't be serious' or 'it can't happen to me' and try to shut it out of their minds. A calm, apparently unruffled demeanour in the midst of crises which would reduce other people to tears or rage or shivering apprehension, can be deceptive. Many such women will probably not even open this book, when they see what it is about, but although we may not be able to change our characters we can be on guard against our weaknesses, or our friends can do it for us.

It is so easy to find 'good' reasons for avoiding something unpleasant, like being too busy, or waiting until after the long-planned family holiday, or convincing yourself that you are making a fuss about nothing. Fear can make cowards or fools of us all and it is not always the case that we react instinctively in our own best interests. It is natural and understandable to fear cancer, but we must not allow that fear to develop into a phobia because if that happens, we are no longer capable of coping rationally. Above all, don't allow yourself to take a fatalistic attitude towards the disease. So many people believe that if they are 'doomed' to get cancer there is nothing they can do about it, and that no treatment can affect the outcome.

This is just not true. Cancer is curable. In Britain alone, it is estimated that some 30,000 people are cured of cancer *every year*, many of them women with either breast or cervical cancer, both conditions with a good prognosis if they are found really early. This brings us to the other diagnostic aids which can be used to examine women's breasts.

At the breast clinic

A GP will see only a very few suspicious breast symptoms during a year's practice and he is not likely, therefore, to be very skilled at palpating breasts unless he has made a point of making this a part of the routine examination of women patients. Neither is he qualified to diagnose cancer so the most he can do is make an intelligent guess about the nature of the symptom. The conscientious doctor will, therefore, recommend a woman to see a specialist, if he finds anything abnormal, however insignificant it may appear to be, on the grounds that it is better to be safe than sorry. This must be your attitude too. Furthermore, it is most important that you are referred to a breast specialist who is backed by all the facilities of a well-equipped breast unit and a medical team. Unfortunately there are not too many of these but for an up-to-date list of NHS breast units, or clinics as they are usually called, see page 141.

Because breast cancer is a relatively common disease, many general surgeons will reckon that they know how to deal with it, but unless they have a reputation for specializing in breast surgery, they probably do no more than a dozen mastectomies a year, if that. This does not qualify them as specialists in a disease which anyway, as we shall see later, cannot be treated adequately with surgery alone. I shall repeat this vital point more than once during the course of this book because until women realize that breast cancer is a complicated disease requiring various complex skills from doctors with different medical specializations working together, they will never get the treatment they need. In my view, our first priority should be for more breast clinics, furnished with all the necessary diagnostic facilities – one attached to every General District Hospital in the country – so that GPs would always know where to send their patients for the best attention. This is at least as important a demand as campaigning for a screening service, which has yet to prove its efficacy. Ideally, one would be complementary to the other and both be based in the same premises, using the same resources.

Let us imagine that you are lucky enough to live near a hospital with a breast clinic, and that your GP knows about it; not always as inevitable as you might think, which is one reason why the list on page 141 may be useful to you. With slight variations, this is what you can expect to happen at a well-run clinic, when you go for your first appointment.

First, you will be *clinically examined* by the surgeon who begins by investigating the breast with the symptom, comparing its appearance with the other one and carefully palpating it, much in the manner that was described in the previous chapter for breast self-examination. His purpose is to find out what sort of lump it is; how large it is; whether it is mobile or fixed; and whether it seems contained or spreading. The general appearance of the breast is also very significant to the experienced clinician. If you have spotted any of those warning signs on your list he will see them too and he will want to know when you first noticed them. If you have delayed coming to the doctor, don't make things worse now by pretending that you have only just discovered them. It is crucially important for him to have all the facts to help him in his diagnosis, so answer all his questions truthfully.

After he has examined the symptomatic breast he will turn his attention to the other and palpate it in the same thorough way. By this time he will have a fairly good idea of what he thinks you have; whether it is some type of benign disease, which it will be nine times out of ten; or whether it could possibly be a malignancy. Some cancers are immediately obvious to the experienced doctor. Unhappily, this is often because the woman has delayed and so it has progressed to a stage which is visibly diagnosable, but it can also be due to the type of cancer – either very fast growing or highly inflamed.

He will not rely on his clinical judgement alone for a diagnosis. You will then be sent to the radiology department to have a *mammogram*, an X-ray technique which has been specially developed for taking pictures of soft fatty tissue. In fact, the larger and therefore the more fatty the breast, the better the picture that will be produced because any lesions in the breast show up vividly against the fat. It is also more difficult for the clinician to find a lump in a big breast because it can be tiny and buried too deep for him to feel with his fingers, so mammography is an essential complementary diagnostic aid. Mammography is less effective for women with small breasts which contain little fat and are probably much denser structures but with these the clinician has a better chance of picking up abnormalities. Xerograms which produce a sharper picture, but do have a slightly higher radiation dose, are also favoured for the dense, small breast. However, when a doctor is looking for a malignancy, as he is with any symptomatic woman who is referred to a breast clinic, this once-only higher dose can be justified.

Another excellent use for mammograms is that the picture may show up other, quite unsuspected abnormalities in another part of the breast or even in the opposite one. This acts as a double check against the surgeon's examination which inadvertently will tend to concentrate on the symptomatic breast.

Some breast units will also do a *thermogram*. This is a completely harmless means of measuring, by infra-red radiation, the varying heat patterns of the body. The breasts are first cooled and then any 'hot spot' which is picked up indicates an abnormality which is not necessarily a malignancy. And this is a major problem about thermograms; they pick up a lot of 'false positives' which on further examination prove to be non-cancerous. Equally, they pick up 'false negatives' which would be even more dangerous if they were not counter-checked by a mammogram.

There are a few enthusiasts who persist with thermography because they believe that it has a special role to play in breast cancer diagnosis. In certain cases where neither mammogram nor clinical examination are conclusive, the thermogram can provide the decisive evidence. About 85 per cent of cancers are hot and the degree of heat tends to be a prognostic indicator in itself. The hotter, the less good the prognosis is. Used consistently, they could also be developed as a useful biological profile. Just as our fingerprints are unique to each of us, so apparently are thermograms and an experienced doctor, picking one up, will immediately recognize it as 'Mrs Jones' or 'Mrs Smith'. The ones to watch over a long period of time are those which are hot but apparently benign. Evidence from one thermographic unit shows that 12 per cent of these 'hot' breasts eventually develop cancer.

Surveys in highly specialized breast units show that the average pick-up rate for accurate diagnosis of cancer is 85 per cent when done by a radiologist reading a mammogram. When surgeon and radiologist work together, their combined accuracy is 98 per cent because each will pick up a few different cases, leaving just one or two out the first time round because both will have mistaken for benign a lesion which on biopsy turns out to be malignant.

A *biopsy* is the removal of a small piece of suspect tissue which will then be sent to the pathologist for analysis. It can be done with a needle as an out-patient procedure or surgically, under a general anaesthetic. If the doctor thinks that you have a cyst – very common in women over 30 and usually very recognizable because it tends to be mobile and feel soft and springy to the touch, rather like a tiny balloon – he will aspirate it there and then. This is a quick, painless procedure requiring no anaesthetic. The doctor plunges a needle into the head of the cyst and draws off the thin, yellowish-coloured fluid which will be sent off for analysis just to make sure that it contains no malignant cells. He will also have the extra precaution of your mammogram to tell him whether there is anything else suspicious in either of your breasts. Nine times out of ten there isn't and you can go home feeling reassured, but don't become over-confident. Cysts have a way of coming back, and back, and they should always be attended to. Meanwhile continue doing your regular monthly breast self-examination.

Should the lump be more solid, then the doctor may decide to do what is called a tru-cut needle biopsy which is also an outpatient procedure. No more painful than an injection, the needle draws out a tiny bit of tissue from the lump which will then go immediately to the laboratory for analysis. This gives the doctor a preliminary idea about the nature of your lump, but at the same time an appointment will be made for you to come into hospital within the next week or so to have a second biopsy under general anaesthetic. Whether the lump is benign or malignant it must come out and the wider cut (excision) this requires could not be done under a local anaesthetic. This is true for all women over the age of 30, when any lump has to be treated with great caution, but some surgeons will make exceptions for very young women who rarely have malignant lumps but do often produce a mimic condition called fibroadenoma which can be removed under local anaesthetic. It too will be sent off for analysis because the unlucky one in a hundred will turn out to be malignant.

For those women who report symptoms other than lumps, the mammogram verdict is very important. Again, regardless of what the doctors privately surmise about the reading, you will have to come in for a biopsy, even if it only serves to confirm the good news that your condition is harmless. This is yet another reason why the mammograph is such a valuable diagnostic aid; it can pick up alterations in the breast some time before they are detectable either by the woman or the clinician. It is undoubtedly our best means yet of picking up really early cancers and its invention has made screening a vital issue, as we shall see in the next chapter.

It is worth repeating that most women will leave the breast clinic reassured that there is nothing seriously wrong with them. However, the model breast clinic will retain what is called a baseline mammograph and, if they have the facility, a thermogram as well. The woman will be asked to attend at regular intervals for a check-up and possibly every three years have another mammogram to compare it with the original. This is a form of screening but it is only available to symptomatic women.

5 To screen or not to screen?

You may be surprised that such a question should even be raised. We may be rather vague in our ideas about what constitutes a good health education programme, or how certain diseases can be prevented rather than cured, but most of us who have thought about the subject at all tend to the view that if screening is possible, then those who have need of it should have right of access to it. Whether they choose to use it is their business. Alas! if only it were so simple, and this is especially true in the case of breast cancer.

The real question that must be asked about screening for any potentially lethal disease is: *does it save lives?* Nothing less than a positive reduction in the mortality figures can justify the vast expense of launching a mass screening programme, but if there is a method of screening which can be proved to save lives, then on ethical grounds alone no government has the right to withhold this service, particularly from any section of the population which is known to be at risk.

Where breast cancer is concerned, this deceptively straightforward question immediately raises other, very thorny issues to which the solutions have not yet been found but which again must be answered before we can demand a national screening service for breast cancer. These are the basic questions which the Department of Health and Social Security has built into its recently launched national screening trials. It will take ten to fifteen years before they yield final answers.

First, even if you prove that finding a cancerous lesion in the breast earlier gives a better chance of survival, can you be certain that the subsequent treatment is adequate?

Second, how do you accurately define a high-risk population and are these the only women to whom you should offer the service?

Third, how do you motivate the women you consider need the service to use it? And how do you educate the doctors to educate them?

Fourth, how sure can you be that your screening techniques are the best? How much time and money can you afford trying them out, or measuring them against alternatives?

Fifth, how much unnecessary anxiety and possibly ill-health (morbidity) are you in danger of provoking?

Sixth, where does an expensive national breast cancer screening programme stand in the scale of priorities as compared with other urgent pressures on an already over-stretched health service?

These are cold, hard questions, the sort that only economists and statisticians and research scientists can answer. They may seem cruelly irrelevant to the human suffering caused by breast cancer, and indeed they are to the individual woman, and her family, who are stuck with it now, but in the cause of long-term improved control of the disease for everyone, the government has no alternative but to wait for conclusive answers.

To date, there has only been one* large-scale screening programme which was deliberately set up as a trial running over many years – started in 1963 – and from which follow-up results are still being culled. This is the famous New York Health Insurance programme, known as the HIP Study, which even those who are its sternest critics concede was brilliantly devised and carried out by its begetters, Shapiro, Strax and Venet. HIP, rather like our BUPA, is a private medical insurance scheme.

Between 1963 and 1969, 62,000 women members, all between the ages of 40 and 64 and all living within the greater New York area, were randomly allocated to one of two groups: 31,000 to the 'study group' who were offered screening for breast cancer and 31,000 to the 'control group' who were not. Screening involved an

*The results of two smaller but more recent European studies (Holland and Sweden) show that better techniques are picking up more cancers which suggests, in the words of the British Breast Group Statement, that 'the potential benefits of screening today may be much larger than those found in the HIP study'.

initial examination which included taking a detailed medical, social and family history, followed by a clinical examination, mammography and thermography. The women were then asked to return for three further annual check-ups. Despite the fact that 10,000 women refused to participate in the study group (one-third) and despite too the inevitable disappearance of women from HIP records after five years (about 20 per cent in both groups), careful follow-up, now approaching the ten-year mark, shows a consistent *one-third reduction in the number of deaths from breast cancer among women aged over 50 in the study group.* In other words, screening is effective, and has been proven beyond doubt, but for post-menopausal women only. What makes it effective is the combination of mammography with clinical examination. (Thermography, as we have seen, tends to be too unreliable to be counted in as a diagnostic aid, although it may have other uses.)

One-third of the cancers picked up were detected by mammography alone, whereas only two-fifths were found solely by clinical examination which is somewhat different from the combined pick-up rate which is normal in a symptomatic examination (see page 40). In addition to proving how necessary it is to use both techniques, this fact also makes a strong case for the value of mammography picking up earlier cancers since 79 per cent of those found by mammography alone were shown to be free of lymph node involvement as compared to 75 per cent found by clinical examination alone. (Lymph node status, as it is called, is an important indication as to whether the disease has advanced and how much.)

Figures, figures, figures, you may be saying impatiently. Everyone knows that they can be used to prove anything. What matters is to save lives and if one-third of the women in Britain today who are over 50 and threatened with breast cancer could have their lives saved by screening, surely that is a price well worth paying? (At the time of writing, the estimated yearly cost of running a full-scale screening programme for women over the age of 45 is £50 million.) The unpleasant contrary argument, but it is one that must be faced because it all boils down to these two things in the end – results and money – is that for every woman you pick up at screening and treat for breast cancer, you spend £5,000; a large sum of money which is diverted from spending on research to improve methods of treatment and discover other more effective means of early detection. This is obviously acceptable if you can also prove that the women you pick up from screening do more than live. *They must live longer because they are cured. The cancer has been caught so early, it has not had a chance to spread.*

This has yet to be proved.

How early is early? This is a problem which still baffles the oncologists, the people who specialize in cancer. Tumour cells grow by doubling. One cancer cell becomes two, then becomes four, eight, sixteen and so on. Some tumours grow rapidly, doubling themselves every few days, others take a year or more, but where it has been possible to measure them, it seems the average doubling rate is somewhere between one and five months. However, not all tumours follow the same pattern so although, broadly speaking, a tiny tumour indicates early disease and a large one indicates advanced disease, a disturbing number of early lesions which are picked up on the mammogram – and this can mean no more than a slight alteration in the tissue – prove, on further investigation, to be already invasive, that is to say the cancer has spread to the lymph nodes.

The smallest tumour a mammogram can pick up is about half a centimetre in size; the smallest tumour a woman or her doctor can pick up is about two centimetres. If you realize that a centimetre of tumour represents one gram of tissue which is about a billion cells, or thirty doubling times, which could have taken anything from three to eight years to grow in what is known as the 'silent interval', the nature of the problem becomes evident. Even at one centimetre, the tumour is unlikely to be symptomatic; at two, it may just be, and at four it obviously will be but the woman will also be potentially very ill.

The fundamental question this poses *vis-à-vis* the advantage of mammography for screening is how many of these early lesions that are picked up, some of which may even be pre-cancerous, belong to a tumour type which disseminates early into the body, sometime during that 'silent interval' period when the tumour has been doubling and doubling and doubling? Lymph node involvement is a 'marker' that tells the doctors the disease has already spread, but unfortunately the reverse is not an invariable negative indication. Doctors believe that in some cases, even when the lymph nodes are unaffected, stray cancer cells have already slipped into the blood circulation. Often these cells are destroyed by the woman's own bodily defences and so may never lead to further trouble, but breast cancer has many forms, some of which are more likely to spread (metastasize). Whatever the type, it is improbable that the spread will be caught in the single doubling time that may occur between mammographic and clinical pick-up.

This is not to say that mammography is not a marvellous diagnostic tool but its effectiveness as a screening technique can only be judged by the number of genuinely early cancers it picks up, that is to say, cancers which are biologically early, rather than just clinically early. Time and systematic investigation alone can give us this important answer.

However, the outlook is optimistic for women over 50 and since increasing age is the most certain high-risk factor, the Department of Health and Social Security, after much consultation, has pitched a large-scale screening trial to involve 240,000 women over the age of 45 in eight different areas of the country. The centres have been matched as closely as possible for demographic features such as class, proportion of urban to rural inhabitants, spread of occupation, etc., but inevitably there are differences, as the critics hasten to point out. Again, time alone will reveal whether they are crucial. As in the HIP study, four of these centres are the 'study groups' and the other four, notable for their altruism because they will get no benefits apart from their names on the subsequent reports, are the comparison centres. Two of the 'study groups' are offering a screening service using the standard procedures of clinical examination, medical history and mammography every other year for seven years with clinical examination alone in the intervening years. The other two centres will be teaching breast self-examination, again to invited groups, but using different methods and different locales. All four centres will then be compared against each other and against the control groups.

No one could accuse the DHSS of rushing into this programme. Before deciding on the final structure they ran three feasibility trials in different parts of the country to test various hypotheses and methods. For instance, one centre concentrated particularly on seeing how well paramedical personnel, people like nurses and radiographers, could be trained to do clinical examinations – palpating breasts – and reading mammograms. Methods of inviting women to participate and noting the most responsive age and class were compared. The pros and cons of the different techniques – thermography, mammography and xeromammography – were carefully weighed; and the difficulties of teaching breast self-examination effectively – and indeed whether it is worthwhile at all – were considered.

At the time of writing, Edinburgh has the only purpose-built National Health Service screening unit in the country, although there will shortly be a second one in the South of England. The unit is staffed entirely by women, including the darkroom technician, most of whom are married, work part-time and are about the same age as the clients. Opened on 1 July 1975, it had examined by August 1978 almost 5,000 women between the ages of 40 and 59 who were invited by a personal letter from their own doctors. Twelve GP practices took part. Screening involved mammograms (which were interpreted independently by two doctors), a detailed medical history (on the first visit), clinical examination by two doctors and, in the earlier months of the project, they had thermography as well, but this technique was finally rejected because the unit was technically unsatisfactory. Examinations and mammograms were repeated at annual intervals for three years. Just under half the cancers (twenty in all) were picked up by mammography alone, and several were picked up by mammography after a first negative clinical finding, which was then repeated and a palpable lesion found, proving that clinical examination combined with mammography is better than either method on its own.

This is a model unit because all the women screened were, apart from their age, invited without any pre-selection; self-referring women who may well be worried by a symptom of some sort are not included in the findings and this is very important in statistical terms, because you can only make an accurate judgement about the value of a screening programme when you offer it to a normally healthy population. The fact that the staff is entirely female is also important. Although I have only seen it acknowledged in one paper, there are undoubtedly many women who are put off and embarrassed by the prospect of having their breasts exposed and manipulated to the extent which is necessary for mammography as well as clinical examination. It is also true that many women find it easier to ask questions of a doctor of their own sex, and maybe confide their worries. For these reasons the preliminary conclusions coming out of this unit are interesting both in themselves and as a guide for those in charge of planning future screening programmes.

First, it had an unexpectedly good response – 82 per cent – from a well mixed population; not only did working-class women come forward in equal numbers with their middle-class sisters but the Clinical Director says that she and her colleagues were impressed by the high level of intelligent, informed comments and questions which they put. This augurs well for the acceptance of a national screening service because as Dr Philip Strax so rightly puts it: 'A screening detection process is only as good as its acceptance by the population at risk,' and in terms of cost-effectiveness, women's response is all important. Second, out of those twenty-odd cancers which were detected, more than half proved to be before lymph node involvement. Again an encouraging sign. Less good is the impression the doctors have that screening can cause a lot of unadmitted alarm in the many women who are diagnosed with benign breast disease and are therefore sent for biopsy. Fear is difficult to measure but it becomes significant if it stops women coming for further checks; vice versa, an all-clear can make a woman feel dangerously self-confident. Finally, a quarter of the cancers were picked up on a second or third screening which poses another problem: how often should a woman be screened to give her really adequate protection? Some would say every year from the age of 40 onwards: others, even those who are most enthusiastic about screening, are more cautious because of the increased radiation risk.

Mammographic techniques are improving all the time and the radiation dose is now a fraction of what was given in the HIP study, but it still is a risk for younger women. As a rough guide women over the age of 50 are relatively safe but no woman under the age of 40 should have a mammogram for other than diagnostic purposes: in other words, unless she presents with a symptom that cannot be satisfactorily diagnosed by clinical examination alone. Under the age of 25 she should not have one for any reason at all because the truly young breast is acutely radiosensitive as all the studies quoted in Chapter 2 show. This means that the tissue is particularly susceptible to the small but unavoidable radiation dose which is contained in any X-ray and can cause cancer. Women considering referring themselves to a privately-run screening unit for a well-woman check-up must bear this in mind.

Making the service as accessible as possible is another important characteristic of an efficient screening programme. It will therefore be interesting to see what response the screening centre in the South of England has with its three mobile vans in rural areas. The health education programmes and invitations to learn breast self-examination which are being run in the other two trial centres are also of immense importance. Although no doctor would openly discourage a woman from doing breast self-examination, many have private reservations about its value, mainly because they suspect that very few women do it in the regular routine way which is essential as I stressed in Chapter 3. The doctor in charge of the hospital-based trial is positive, however, that if women can only be persuaded to do it properly, they have a very good chance of picking up lumps before the clinician can. He is supported in this view by the man with the longest experience anyone has of running a screening service, Dr Philip Strax, who, reporting in 1976 on the previous five-year period of his screening service, said that 'the importance of teaching breast self-examination is highlighted by finding about nine per cent "interval" cancers with 66 per cent no nodal involvement.' These are the cancers which appear suddenly between examinations and without any warning on the previous mammogram.

All in all, the DHSS will have a lot to think about when eventually it comes to weighing up the pros and cons of providing a national screening service. Meanwhile, research is continuing into alternative, easier, cheaper and more definitive methods of detecting early breast cancer, some of which are discussed later in this book. Our best hope is that the present somewhat ponderous screening trials will be overtaken by events because somebody will have hit on the simple safe test everybody is looking for to offer to high-risk women.

part two

Action

6 A change of mind

Ten years ago there were one or two voices in the wilderness suggesting that the time had come for a fundamental re-evaluation of the nature of breast cancer. Today, there is a massively growing chorus of support for such a view, backed by convincing evidence, and this significant change of opinion is reflected in new concepts about how the disease should be treated. At this stage of research, there are still many questions requiring an answer and many problems awaiting a solution, but certain facts have been established.

First, breast cancer is not one single type of disease. Not only does it present itself in different ways, as we have seen by the variety of symptoms for which we should be on the look-out, but it behaves in different ways and this is because breast cancer tumours are biologically diverse, one from another.

Second, breast cancer is not necessarily located in one single site, the breast. It starts there, but by the time it is discovered, even when apparently very early, it may already have released cancer cells into the blood stream which have circulated and settled in distant parts of the body, starting up new cancer sites which may be so minute that they are quite undetectable and for a long time produce no symptoms. These are called micro-metastases. It is now believed, mainly on the basis of ten-year survival figures, but there is other evidence as well, that approximately 80 per cent of breast cancers have already disseminated into other parts of the body before they are picked up.

Third, it is now recognized that although the degree of lymph node involvement is an important prognostic indication for the outcome of the disease, it is not the only one. Furthermore, an absence of tumour in the lymph nodes does not necessarily signify that the disease is confined to the breast.

Fourth, whichever of the traditional methods for locally

treating the disease is chosen, that is to say, surgery or radio-therapy, or a combination of both, where the aim is to remove the tumour in the breast, it has been proved, again by the figures, that none of them makes any difference in terms of survival. Survival depends on the nature of the tumour which biologically pre-determines the final outcome. This is not to say that surgery does not make an essential contribution to controlling the disease, but it can no longer be regarded as the only definitive way of produc-ing a cure.

The combined effect of these very telling facts produces the following conclusions: breast cancer is almost invariably a sys-temic disease which should, therefore, be treated systemically. Just as the disease itself is not a single entity, so there is no single way of treating it. But conclusions don't produce answers. Those who are most experienced in the treatment of breast cancer agree that a pooling of different skills and different disciplines offers the only hope of finding the right method of treatment for the individual woman. This is called the multi-disciplinary or com-bined modality approach but how the various therapies should be combined, and to what degree, and when, are still matters for research. Answers are being urgently sought in the enormous number of breast cancer trials which are currently going on all over the world.

Amidst so much uncertainty there is only one certainty – the truly knowledgeable know how much they still don't know, even if they have some very promising theories – so beware the claim of anyone who is supposed to have the answer to breast cancer. On the other hand, it is unwise to consult someone who has not got a special interest in breast cancer because it is a disease which enlists a wide range of medical specializations. Epidemiology, surgery, endocrinology, radiology, oncology, pathology, pharma-cology and psychology are all required, so it follows that the best that can be offered today in the way of treatment will only be available in those hospitals which have a breast unit run by a medical team able to call on all these areas of expertise. We British are fortunate because we can find these facilities within the National Health Service; admittedly, not yet enough of them, but by exerting some pressure we could have more, and where they do exist they are first-rate. My advice to any woman needing treatment for any breast problem, whether it proves to be benign or malignant, is to ask her GP to send her to her nearest breast unit (see list on page 141). There she can be certain of receiving the best available treatment, *immediately*, which is most important and, equally valuable, she will be assured of careful, long-term follow-up attention which is not always guaranteed with private treatment. It is nice to be positive about our much-abused (on the whole unfairly) National Health Service. Here is an example of its immeasurable advantage over systems of medical care in many other countries where it is not unknown for desperate women to hawk around their breast cancers from one doctor to the next until they find one who is unscrupulous enough to do what they want, which may not be what they need.

While it is the purpose of this book to give the reader as much information as possible about breast cancer so that she knows what to expect and what it may involve, my second piece of advice to any woman who finds she does need treatment, is to accept what is prescribed, having once made her choice of hospital and always providing, of course, that it seems reasonable to her. Obviously, this does not mean that she should stop asking questions. On the contrary, she should ask as often and as many questions as she likes and she will find that most doctors and nurses will respond gladly. Furthermore, no one will oblige her to accept a particular treatment if she objects strongly enough, but, generally speaking, it is sensible to accept the advice of the doctors in charge, bearing in mind their considerable experience in treating the disease and their unfaltering dedication to the cause of doing the best they can for each one of their patients. Trust between doctor and patient is an important constituent of recovery in the management of any illness. In the case of breast cancer, you must be satisfied that you understand the reason behind the doctor's choice of a particular therapy. After that, leave it to them.

Unfortunately, and for a number of reasons, the discussion of which are irrelevant to this book, although they are extremely pertinent to the overall future of the National Health Service, not all hospitals can offer equally high standards in terms of quality of staff, flexibility of treatment and up-to-date equipment. This provides yet another strong argument for campaigning for more breast units but as far as this book is concerned there seems little advantage in looking at the worst side of things. The remainder of Part Two, therefore, examines the new theories about breast cancer in more detail because they are having a fundamental influence on methods of treatment. It also describes the best action for a diagnosed breast cancer which a woman can expect to receive today in a model breast unit, action which is based on the new thinking.

7 What are they looking for?

As a first step we should accept the idea that
breast cancer is a systemic disease until proved otherwise
(The Curability of Breast Cancer, Michael Baum, 1977)

This view, expressed by one of our leading younger surgeons in a recent contribution to a book on the treatment of breast cancer (written for doctors), is not exclusive to him, as he would certainly agree, but it is taking a long time to gain general acceptance and among older, more conservative medical circles it is still considered to be somewhat radical. That it comes from a surgeon is especially interesting, because traditionally it is this branch of the profession which has master-minded the management of breast cancer and has been jealous of any attempts to suggest that other forms of treatment have anything but a minor role to play. The more you cut, the better the chances of cure, has been the consistent philosophy of most surgeons from the days of Halsted on, but more about all that in Chapter 8.

However, to be fair to the distinguished dissenting minority, Michael Baum is by no means alone among his kind. Indeed, much of the most advanced thinking about new ways of tackling breast cancer comes from the surgeons themselves, those more reflective ones who have looked at the distressing lack of improvement in the mortality figures over the past thirty years, despite improved techniques of surgery, radiotherapy and anaesthesia, and who have asked themselves why. Slowly, it has been borne in on them that women who get it are not necessarily lucky to have it in a part of their body which can be lopped off easily without causing excessive physical damage. (The idea that such an amputation might cause psychological injury is even more recent in origin and is taking even longer to penetrate, but that too is reserved for discussion in Chapter 12.)

The major reason for knowing that breast cancer has often spread before it is diagnosed are the survival figures. No woman who has had breast cancer wants to think of herself as a survival statistic. And rightly too! The way to make the most of the life we have, and this applies to everyone, not just those who have had cancer, is to live every day as it comes. Flipping over the calendar pages and marking off each year you survive is a life-denying and unnatural exercise. However, it is a different matter for doctors in their professional capacity as healers. They must look at the survival figures dispassionately if they are to read them correctly, so 5, 10 and 15 years have become significant beacons for judging cure rates. And some very important long-term studies are extending these figures to 20 and 25 years.

The traditional view of the disease made it a simple, clear-cut forecast based on the following mechanistic principles. It was believed that breast cancer developed in stages. First, it appeared in the breast where it stayed for some time, then it moved to the lymph nodes which act as immune filters in the body's drainage system and where again it would slowly spread. If the tumour was found and removed before it had reached the lymph nodes, then the woman was cured. If only one or two involved lymph nodes were found then the woman's chances of permanent cure were slightly reduced but if the spread was considerable, then her chances were drastically diminished. It is certainly true that extensive lymph node involvement is a sign that the disease has spread and broken through the lymph node barrier, but what truly confounds the theory that breast cancer progresses through these ordered stages is the fact that two-thirds of the women who do not have any lymph node involvement at the time of their operation do not survive beyond fifteen years. Furthermore, it has been known in a significant number of cases for the disease to reappear more than twenty years after the first diagnosis.

These facts strongly suggest that cutting out the tumour does not always dispose of the entire malignancy. In Chapter 5 I described the way a tumour grows and that there is a long 'silent interval' when it is continually doubling itself. There is considerable evidence to show that a tumour is most active in its early stages, and that by the time it has been discovered it has probably reached a plateau stage where, because it is essentially a disordered organism, it may be losing more old cells than it is growing new ones, with the result that the doubling time slows down. In its active period, however, experiments show that it is likely to have shed a considerable number of live cells, 'seeding' as the process is sometimes called, some of which will be killed by the body's defence mechanisms, but others of which are likely to have escaped, bypassing the lymph nodes entirely and lying dormant for years until some change in the body reactivates them. There is also a new theory that lymph nodes are not quite as effective a barrier as had originally been thought and that instead of regarding positive or negative nodes as an indication of whether the disease has spread or not, we should assume that breast cancer always disseminates itself. If this is so, then negative nodes show that they have done a good job of killing off the seeded cells, whereas positive nodes indicate that either they have not been able to cope with the particular biological type of tumour – remember there are different types of breast cancer – or that there were too many malignant cells for them to destroy.

If this theory is correct, then it supports the view that no-node involvement at the time of diagnosis makes a good prognosis but it also explains why the prognosis is not always confirmed in the long run. It is not a question of waiting to see whether the cancer will return because on this theory the cancer *has never gone away*. It assumes that it is present in other parts of the body, almost from the start of the tumour's development, certainly long before it is discovered, and if this is so it also explains why surgery does not always ensure a cure, even in the most hopeful cases.

At first reading, this may seem an alarming, utterly depressing theory. If we must accept that breast cancer is nearly always, by the time it is discovered, systemic, then what hope is there for finding a total cure? It is no surprise that many doctors, particularly surgeons whose life work has been based on doing radical, that is to say extensive, surgery for breast cancer, are reluctant to accept it, but unless the new generation does, the much more terrible outlook is that there will be no change in the mortality figures for the next thirty years. In fact, it is an exciting and hopeful theory based on a growing body of evidence and it opens up entirely new vistas on the way the disease should be handled. This starts at the moment when a woman visits a breast clinic for the first time and a malignancy is suspected.

A second visit to the breast clinic

We take up now from the point where we left off at the end of Chapter 4 to follow the one woman in five whose lump does require further investigation. The procedures which are described vary in detail from clinic to clinic but basically they follow the same principle: a programme of treatment can only be decided after making as thorough an investigation as possible. This means that if there is a suspicious abnormality, which may or not have been partially confirmed by a needle biopsy at that first visit, an appointment will now be made for her to come into hospital within the week to have a second more searching biopsy under a general anaesthetic. Guy's Hospital in London has the oldest established breast unit in the country (over forty years) and it is on their long experience that other hospitals have modelled their units so let us see what would happen here.

The new patient clinic is held on Friday afternoons. Those women for whom a biopsy is required are asked to come in on the following Monday morning to a completely separate unit in the hospital which is run by two experienced ward sisters and has the atmosphere of a private wing. Preliminary tests are made and then all these patients have their biopsy on Wednesday morning. Having a biopsy involves a minor operation under general anaesthetic. The surgeon removes a small piece of tissue from the suspect area of the breast which is then immediately frozen – to avoid tissue changes – and raced down to the pathology laboratory for dissection and diagnosis.

In this hospital there is no question of a woman automatically signing a consent form agreeing to a frozen section to be followed by an immediate mastectomy if the verdict is malignant, and this too is an example which is being followed by many other hospitals. It was noticeable in the course of my interviews that the younger surgeons were particularly keen on this. As one said, 'I don't like the idea of putting a whole lot of women to sleep and telling them you may or may not wake up with a breast.'

Humanitarian considerations aside, there are also sound medical reasons for not always relying on a frozen section alone. There are certain conditions which are difficult to diagnose definitely in the ten minutes that a pathologist has to dissect the frozen specimen while the surgeon – and patient – wait in the operating theatre. Furthermore, the type of tumour very often determines the type of operation and the surgeon may want to have the more detailed results which come from submitting the specimen to a paraffin test before making his final decision. Some cancers are of course immediately obvious and in such cases it can be argued that it is more cruel to submit the woman to the anguish of two operations.

Some women would always prefer to rely on the frozen section verdict on the grounds that if there is something wrong it is better to get it over with as quickly as possible; others would not. All women should know, therefore, that the right to make this vital decision rests with them. Even in those hospitals where extensive pre-operative investigations are not carried out, the woman has a right to ask to know the results of her biopsy before agreeing to a mastectomy. It used to be thought that it was highly dangerous to open a cancerous site twice and this was another reason for allowing no delay between biopsy and mastectomy but this too is no longer general medical opinion.

How the biopsy is done is another matter for discussion among surgeons. Some prefer to do as wide an excision as possible in order to be sure that they have extracted all the suspect tissue which may mean removing as much as one quarter of the woman's breast leaving her with heavy scarring and possibly a deformed outline. Others take the opposite view and go to immense lengths to remove as little tissue as possible at this first stage because their aim is to inflict the least deformity that is compatible with safe surgery. Removing a tiny amount of breast tissue through a minute incision requires great skill from the surgeon, but only the best and most experienced will trust themselves to do it and they will follow it up with an X-ray to double-check that they have removed the right piece of tissue.

At Guys, the biopsy results usually come through the following day and, if they show an all-clear, the woman goes home on the Friday. Sometimes, however, the results will take longer because the section is difficult to analyse and requires very careful searching; another argument, in my view, for not relying on frozen section biopsy alone.

The woman who is told that her biopsy has revealed a malignancy will then be told that she must undergo further tests to determine what stage the disease has reached and, if it has spread, to what part of her body. Her lungs will already have been checked. Now she will be given a bone scan – both areas of the body where breast cancer tends to spread first – and her liver will also be tested although this particular test is not yet very reliable. Her blood and urine will also be put through several tests, not so much to determine treatment, but to be banked with similar information from other patients in order to amass evidence which will be used to assist doctors in the future to make more accurate predictions. These tests for staging, as they are called, still need to be improved for completely accurate results, but they do provide a useful guideline for treatment.

In this hospital, as in some others – and they are the best, I can say unequivocally – there is a growing awareness of the psychological suffering that this particular disease brings with it and later I shall describe some of the things a few, but not nearly enough, hospitals are doing to help women before and after mastectomy. Some doctors rely on their nurses to counsel the patients; others will try and do it themselves, more or less well, as the most honest among them ruefully admit. Most are agreed, however, that the patient has a right to the truth, but how that truth is told is another problem. If the condition is definitely malignant, then it is wrong to tell her that 'it is on the turn' or use some other euphemism which deep down deceives no one, least of all the woman herself. People are different, however, and some will prefer not to ask, or even say to the doctor, when he may try to explain, words to the effect that she doesn't want to know the details. She trusts him to do the right thing.

However, people reading this book are likely to be of a more inquiring and persistent frame of mind. They are reading it because they want to know the truth about the disease and they will want to know the truth about themselves. Again I can only repeat that in the best hospitals, if you ask questions you will be given truthful answers.

Many women might think that this week of investigation and uncertainty would increase their anxiety and create an almost unbearable situation. However, many who have experienced it say that sharing their crisis with other women in the same situation made them feel more prepared to accept their subsequent treatment and it also helped them to cope, which may sound surprising but it has been confirmed to me over and over again. This is also the opinion of Dr Maureen Roberts in Edinburgh who has been in charge of such a clinic for many years and who has always been deeply concerned about the patient's involvement. In her unit, the women are free to come and go as they like, providing they keep their appointments. They get up and dress in their own clothes in the morning like normal people, go out shopping, meet friends for coffee and meanwhile they can talk about their situation, confide in each other or the nurses, get to know the doctors and generally by the end of the week the urgency and desperation has gone out of the situation. Dr Roberts admits that she can't prove anything because she has not done a controlled study on it, but her feeling, which is shared by the rest of the hospital staff, is that on the whole most women become calmer and more accepting as the week goes on. If the verdict is that an operation is necessary, this still comes as a shock, but they have at least the confidence that the hospital staff has done and will continue to do everything which is in the best interest of their patients.

Breast cancer is a matter of urgency. Treating it must not be delayed, but one week between diagnosis and operation, if that is what ultimately proves to be necessary, is not going to make any difference at all. And if that week means that a woman has been given a chance to face up to what is ahead, and to summon the reserves of strength she will undoubtedly need, then it seems to me to be an infinitely preferable course of action to the traditional scenario of diagnosis one day, bundling into hospital the next day, and waking up on the third without a breast. Mastectomy, in any circumstances, is a trauma; under those conditions, it seems to me positively barbaric and I believe should not be tolerated by women any longer.

8 Is your operation really necessary?

A few years ago that question would have been unthinkable in any group of doctors concerned with the treatment of breast cancer. Today it is regarded as heresy only by the most orthodox. The more open-minded and scientifically biased members of the profession are considering it with cautious interest and there is a growing conviction among the present generation of specialists in the field that there is a reasonable hope for the future that the majority of women will both be able to keep their breasts and receive better, that is to say more effective, treatment for their cancer. When that day will come is still anybody's guess and depends on the outcome of current trials going on in all the major world centres of breast cancer research which are comparing different regimes of what is called adjuvant therapy. As the name suggests, this is therapy applied in conjunction with the primary surgery and it aims to attack the cancer globally, throughout the body, on the assumption that it has probably disseminated by the time it has been diagnosed. Hormone therapy and chemotherapy listed in the order of their historical appearance as therapeutic agents, are the two major arms of this attack and how they are being used is described in more detail in Chapter 10.

Women, of course, have always asked this question and been dismissed as hysterical or foolish or both – a familiar response which they know only too well in many other areas of their life but one to which they have become less and less amenable. While I am not suggesting that the present resurgence of the women's movement, which is slowly making its mark in the whole area of health care, has been especially influential in changing attitudes about surgical treatment of breast cancer, I do believe that its revival during this last decade has been a precipitating factor. It is not just pure coincidence that at a time when women are becoming much more demanding and much less accepting, the medical profession – always a strong authoritarian element in women's lives – is hastening to reappraise its management of breast cancer.

After all, the grim facts have been staring doctors in the face for more than half a century; to wit, however they wield the knife it makes no difference in the end. The same appallingly high number of women have been dying every year with advanced breast cancer which may return 10, 15, 20 or even more years after its first appearance. While there were no alternatives to surgery obviously little could be done, except to improve the selection of cases for operation, and indeed, when this was realized in the 1940s there was, for a while, a spurious impression of improvement. More women who had a mastectomy began to live longer because only those with a reasonable chance of cure, in other words, those who presented with an early stage cancer, had the operation. But after an initial bump down of the mortality figures they stuck again at the level quoted in Chapter 2 and nothing has budged them since. Sooner or later the questions had to be asked: what are we missing? what else can we try? And now that those questions have been asked and action is being taken to answer them the future looks infinitely more encouraging.

Just as I would not say that women's voices have had more than a marginal effect on this new impetus I also do not subscribe to the view that some surgeons take a sado-chauvinistic pleasure in hacking off women's breasts, even those who are blindly committed to performing the most radical surgery. However, I do confess that my faith in every surgeon's total integrity has been shaken momentarily when I realize the deformity that extended radical surgery entails (not now done in this country); and again when I read how one surgeon as recently as 1965 could describe a woman's breast as 'an affliction of a superficial, easily disposable utilitarian appendage'.* We can only regard these exceptions as the dinosaurs of their profession who are even now, like those ancient monsters, shambling on their way to extinction because their brains are too small to cope with new knowledge. It is not

*T. A. Watson, The Janeway Lecture, 1965, published in the *American Journal of Roentgenology*, Vol 96, (1966), p. 548.

malice which has prompted them to repeat the same useless operation but sheer ignorant prejudice, a refusal to face facts and, it has to be said, sometimes a gross insensitivity to the feelings of their women patients.

As things are, surgery is still necessary for the majority of breast cancers and, in most of those cancers, mastectomy is the best that can be offered to a woman. This is so, even when the doctor suspects that the disease may have spread because he can feel palpable lymph nodes under the arm or there are other adverse signs. Remember that the extent of spread is something which can only be measured, and, even then, not altogether accurately, in those few breast units which are fully equipped with diagnostic machinery. The procedures described in the last chapter are model ones which are not yet available to everyone, unfortunately.

Meanwhile, the usual procedure for most women with a suspicious lump is clinical investigation, which means a visual and manual examination by a general surgeon, followed by biopsy under general anaesthetic to inspect it further, frozen section and then, either simple removal of the lump if it is pronounced benign, or a mastectomy if the verdict is unfavourable.

Clinical staging

When the doctor does his clinical examination he makes a preliminary judgement about the type of cancer and its degree of advancement which is called clinical staging. First he assesses the tumour – its size, whether it is mobile or fixed, whether it feels inflamed. Then he feels the nodes under both arms and surrounding the breasts, to see whether they are enlarged and, if they are, whether they are mobile or fixed. However, nodes, like other lumps in the breast, can be deceptive. They can swell and go down again without any sinister reason and it is for this reason that most doctors are wary of making a definite diagnosis on the basis of clinical staging alone. If he has the facilities, he will then make a further check for metastases doing an X-ray of the chest and certain bones. *Clinical stage one* cancer is defined thus: T1 (tumour under 2 centimetres) or T2 (tumour no larger than 5 centimetres) NO (no palpable nodes) and MO (no evidence of spread beyond the breast). *Clinical stage two* cancer is T1 or T2, N1 (nodes can be felt but they are mobile which is always a better sign) and MO. *Clinical stage three* cancer means that the disease is locally spread so the tumour is large, either T3 (between 5 and 10 centimetres) or T4 (more than 10 centimetres) and several nodes may be felt together with a certain amount of swelling (N2 or N3). *Clinical stage four* is tumour and nodes at any stage combined with evidence of spread to other parts of the body.

Stages one and two are regarded as curable by surgery because the growth seems to be confined to the breast and immediately surrounding tissue. Until much more is known about how and when the disease spreads and, much more important, doctors have alternative proven methods of combating it on a systemic basis, they have really no alternative but to do the orthodox treatment which is a mastectomy, and a woman when she is confronted with this diagnosis would do well to accept the doctor's advice. However, the most a doctor can do is to urge her strongly to accept his recommendation and give her his reason for making it. A woman cannot be forced to have a mastectomy against her will but if she is reluctant she should know the following facts.

First, a tumour that is left will grow, become painful and, worst of all, begin to ulcerate until, if it is left long enough, it becomes an ugly fungating mass, a condition as nasty and smelly as the word suggests which is eventually irreversible. Doctors don't like to warn their patients of this possibility, but in fairness to them and in the pursuit of truth which this book aims to be about, women should appreciate the seriousness of this risk. Local disease is the name given to the area of malignancy which is confined to the breast and axillary nodes. Not only does it spread if it is neglected but it sometimes come back, even after a mastectomy. The reason is that small deposits of cancer cells are left in the skin which, in due course, usually within three years of the original operation, stir into action. This kind of recurrence can, however, be dealt with adequately and swiftly by a short course of radiotherapy.

The second reason for doing a complete rather than a partial mastectomy – this differentiation to be explained – is that breast cancer, in addition to all its other complications, is very often multicentric. What this means is that, apart from the primary tumour, there may be one or more other lesions in the breast which are not advanced enough to be discovered clinically, or even mammographically, but are revealed in the biopsy. No one yet knows how to regard these minor lesions; whether they will regress naturally or whether removal of the primary tumour would precipitate their growth, but in the present state of knowledge it is a legitimate worry for surgeons that, by doing an incomplete mastectomy, they would be leaving behind other potential malignancies.

Which operation?

How complete is complete? This vital question neatly leads us into the next controversial subject regarding breast cancer surgery. Given that an operation is necessary, which one is the best? The surgeon has one aim: he wants to give his patient the best possible chance of cure and depending largely on his personal preference he has five different mastectomy options to choose from, listed here in descending order of size: extended radical, classical radical (Halsted), modified radical, total (or simple), and partial (or lumpectomy).

The *extended radical* involves removing all the breast tissue, both the minor and the major chest muscles, the fat and axillary nodes and *en bloc* removal of the internal mammary nodes which usually means cutting some ribs as well. This operation is never done in this country but it has enthusiastic proponents in the United States including the surgeon who operated on Happy Rockefeller. The justification for doing it is that when a tumour is located on the inner side of the breast, the mammary nodes are almost invariably invaded to which the only comment can be: So What! Why lock the stable door after the horse has bolted? If there is invasion here, it is obvious that the cancer has spread into the body and alternative therapy combined probably with lesser surgery is required, but not this mutilating operation, the effects of which are very difficult for a woman to conceal. She will have a hollow under her arm and be almost concave where her breast and chest wall have been removed.

The *classical radical* (Halsted, so-called, because of the surgeon who invented it eighty-odd years ago) is only slightly less drastic and only slightly less deforming. Everything, except for the mammary nodes, is removed as for the extended radical. A diminishing number of British surgeons perform this operation, mainly of the old school who are unlikely to describe themselves as being especially interested in breast cancer. In America, however, it has an enthusiastic following where it is far and away the operation of choice among surgeons (77 per cent) and it is the most widely practised type of mastectomy throughout the world. The same comment about its effectiveness applies as for the extended radical.

The *modified radical* is a technique which clears the axillary nodes under the arm but preserves the pectoral muscles, thus considerably reducing the external deformity. There is no hollow beneath the shoulder blades and if the scar runs transversely a woman can wear a normal low-necked dress without fear of it showing. In expert hands it is a very good operation and it does almost totally eliminate the chance of local recurrence without having to have post-operative radiotherapy. However, in common with the other radical operations, it can produce the long-term side effect of lymphoedema in the arm on the affected side (heavy arm). This becomes swollen with fluid which can't drain away because the lymphatic system has been removed and in severe cases it can be extremely painful and disabling. It is reckoned that nearly half the patients who have a radical operation will suffer this complication.

The *total* (*or simple*) mastectomy, both misleading names in my view, describe the operation which is becoming increasingly popular in this country, with or without post-operative radiotherapy. It involves removing all the breast tissue, including the tail of the breast but leaving the pectoral muscles and the axillary nodes intact. The argument against this operation is immediately obvious. If you don't remove the axillary nodes how can you judge whether the disease has spread? To which Professor Pat Forrest of Edinburgh has produced an interesting solution. He has devised a technique which is now being copied by many other surgeons where he samples two or three pectoral nodes and also some nodes from the axillary tail. That is to say, at the time of the operation he carefully dissects out these nodes and sends them to the pathologist. He maintains that providing the mastectomy is total, that is to say all the necessary breast tissue is removed, and the surgeon successfully identifies these pectoral nodes in particular, then you can be guided by their condition – whether or not they show signs of tumour spread – in the same way that you can judge spread of disease by counting the involved lymph nodes in the axilla. Various trials are going on at the moment to test the validity of this thesis. The advantage of this operation is that it is less traumatic and less deforming than the radical, there are fewer post-operative complications like arm lymphoedema, but if you don't have post-operative radiotherapy you do run a 30 per cent chance of getting local recurrence. Depending on his bias, a doctor will say that such recurrence can easily be dealt with or shake his head rather gloomily.

Finally there is *partial mastectomy* variously known as *tylectomy, lumpectomy, local* or *wedge* excision. As the name suggests it involves removing the lump and any surrounding affected tissue only. In the past this was considered a disastrous operation, as indeed was the simple mastectomy, but in recent years it has attracted renewed interest, partly because it has offered doctors a chance to give women a less mutilating operation, backed up by radiotherapy to eliminate any malignancy which might have been left behind. Several trials have been run to compare this operation with more radical procedures, one of the best known being a carefully randomized ten-year trial at Guys. Here they discovered that those women with a stage one cancer did as well long-term after a lumpectomy as after a radical. However, if their cancer had progressed to stage two, then both in terms of later metastatic disease and ultimate survival, the women who had had a lumpectomy invariably did less well. Furthermore, many more of those patients who apparently, on clinical examination, had uninvolved nodes got local recurrence, despite their post-operative radiotherapy. The trouble with clinical staging is that it is highly inaccurate when it comes to judging the state of the axillary nodes (about 30 to 40 per cent rate of error) which is significant for the woman whose operation is confined to a lumpectomy, or if she has a simple mastectomy where the surgeon does not employ Professor Forrest's technique.

On the other hand, there are some surgeons who believe that even if you do know that the nodes are involved, the results of long-term trials like the famous 25-year one run jointly by Dr Diane Brinkley at King's College Hospital, London, and Dr John Haybittle at Addenbrooke's Hospital in Cambridge show that ultimately no variation in technique makes any difference in survival. If the disease is there, it will appear again sooner or later, so what everyone should be concentrating on is how to stop it coming back. Meanwhile why do a big operation when you can get away with a little one and reduce the mutilation? The logic of this argument is hard to resist and I am inclined to agree with it. Everybody I have talked to and the innumerable papers I have read produce sound arguments and convincing results to support their favourite operation but even those most in favour of radical surgery are prepared to concede that breast cancer should be treated according to its proven extent. It is in that little word 'proven' that the nub of it all lies and is as yet unsolved. Clinical staging is a guide to prognosis, no more; it is too unreliable to be classed as final proof for any course of treatment. Histologic analysis which involves the minute examination and classification of all the affected organic tissue, is still not completely accurate, but this is a continuing and promising area of research. Another is finding biochemical 'markers' in the body chemistry which indicate the presence of tumours somewhere in the body, but up to now they have been no more precise than that. However, the research currently going on in this field does look very hopeful.

In presenting the different operations I am aware that personal bias has slipped into my description of them. I admit that I believe that the operations at either end of the scale should be avoided; classical and extended radicals because the mutilation they impose

is too great a price to pay for no better results; and the lumpectomy is equally doubtful for the opposite reason – too little
probably too late. However, this operation is correct in certain
cases, for instance, on old women with a slow-growing tumour
who should not be subjected to a big operation. However, as far
as the modified radical and the simple are concerned, I don't
believe there is enough difference between them to worry. In the
hands of a skilled surgeon both yield equally good results cos-
metically and minimal post-operative difficulties, so my advice
would be as before: leave the decision to the surgeon at the breast
unit.

9 A new hope

The surgeon wants, above everything, to give his patient the best possible chance of cure, and for most women with breast cancer, that hope still lies in a mastectomy. However, if he is a sensitive person, he is aware that preservation of life is not enough; it is also important to be able to offer his patient a good quality of life, something that measures up as nearly as possible to what she was enjoying before her illness. The very fact of having a mastectomy, in addition to all its other implications and emotional consequences, serves as a constant reminder to a woman that her life and her body can never again be exactly what they once were. The most well-adjusted woman, whatever her age and circumstances, is bound to feel impaired and damaged, but for some women this sense of mutilation is so strong that it far outweighs their relief at being alive. As a result they can become severely depressed and even mentally ill. Others delay seeking treatment until it is too late because they are so appalled by the thought of the operation.

Until recently, surgeons have not been able to offer any improvement on a mastectomy so, as a measure of self-defence which is understandable but not helpful to their patients, they have tended to dismiss any signs of post-mastectomy psychological disturbance as natural but nothing to worry about. Of course, it's upsetting, they will say, but what's losing one breast as against losing your life? and go on to add that in their experience their patients always recover their emotional stability in the end. Reasonable enough as an argument but not reassuring to the many women who continue to find it very difficult to accept their mutilation. Doctors have been able to delude themselves that their patients are not unduly disturbed by the operation because, quite naturally, few women are willing to expose their unhappiness to someone they instinctively feel is afraid to show them sympathy, especially as they also know that there is nothing else he can do for them and that he has done the best he can.

A few doctors, who have not been so convinced by their patients' apparent stoicism, have been looking at new ways of improving this quality of life, among them better psychological follow-up and therapy if necessary, and also alternative methods of treatment. However, the one to be described now relates entirely to the surgeon's speciality.

For some years, subcutaneous mastectomies followed by implants have been done for certain women with acute benign disease, but recently a few doctors are starting to do them also for women with breast cancer. Subcutaneous means under the skin and implant, or prosthesis, is the name for the artificial breast which is inserted after the breast tissue has been removed.

The operation has three stages. First, the surgeon makes a careful incision, preferably on the underside of the breast so that the scar will eventually be hardly visible, but this is not always possible if the tumour is in an awkward place. He then cuts out all the breast tissue except for a tiny piece under the nipple to hold it in its correct position. Next he matches the false breast against the natural breast for size and shape and this may mean trying several different ones. These days, the prosthesis is made of a soft, malleable absolutely safe silicone gel which is contained in a thin transparent skin, also silicone material. There is absolutely no risk that this substance will leak into other parts of the body or produce any other harmful effects, but it does have one drawback in that it tends to form, after a time, a shell encrustation which somewhat distorts the shape of the breast. However, in such cases it can be removed and a new one inserted. The final stage of the operation comes when the surgeon closes the skin flaps over the implant and sews them up. The patient returns to the ward with the expectation of making as speedy a recovery as any other woman who has had a mastectomy with the one difference that in her two-week post-operative period she may not remove her bandages or start any exercising.

It is estimated that about 15 per cent of the mastectomies performed in Britain every year are for women with benign disease and a certain number of these patients will be getting implants, so surgeons have a good deal of practice in the operation. However, many have been hesitant to offer it to women with breast cancer for fear of possible complications, either arising from the presence of a foreign body brought into contact with tissue which has been disturbed by malignancy or because they feared that if the disease recurred in the breast, it might not be possible to deal with it adequately, for example with radiotherapy.

However, one British surgeon has been doing this implant surgery for twenty years for women with breast cancer and is now producing some very impressive results. I have seen a few of his patients myself and in some of them it was impossible to distinguish the natural breast from the one with the implant. Others do not look perfect – for instance, it is not always possible to preserve the nipple – but inside a bra there is absolutely no difference and he finds that the effect on the women's morale is enormously good. A leader in more ways than one, he was first prompted to try this cosmetic surgery when he realised the extent of the devastating depression many women feel after a mastectomy. He is now recognized as a world authority on this type of surgery, although he is ruefully aware that many of his more conservative British colleagues regard him with suspicion. They suggest that he is not sufficiently academic in writing up his results and that they don't stand up to objective scientific assessment because he only selects the best cases for treatment. I am not qualified to offer any opinion on the first count, except to say that what I have read seems to me to be scrupulously precise. As to the second objection, it is certainly true that he only selects those patients with whom he thinks he has a good chance of success, but it also seems to me that he is perfectly justified in doing this in a situation where what matters above all to the woman herself is her visible external appearance. Providing that the surgeon does not lose sight of his overriding aim which is to effect a cure, then if he can produce this secondary benefit as well, he should surely try it. The surgeon in question is very emphatic on this point. Furthermore, he usually only does this operation for patients with stage one or stage two cancer and it is interesting that in a series of 200 patients on which he has written a paper, only eight of these women later required radiotherapy for local recurrence which he has demonstrated can be done perfectly satisfactorily with the prosthesis remaining in place.

There are also disadvantages to the operation which he is the first to admit. A pronounced change in weight, for example, will affect the size of the natural breast and so cause an obvious discrepancy between it and the one with an implant. Sometimes he can't match the natural breast for technical reasons such as there not being enough skin on the side of the amputated breast but he finds that on the whole his patients are happier with something rather than nothing. He says: 'They want to be able to wear a bikini without embarrassment and try on dresses in a shop without the assistant being able to spot something different.' They also want to be able to undress in front of their husbands and wear low-necked dresses which show a natural cleavage. Sometimes, to counteract the problem of matching, he will do a second operation on the natural breast, especially if it has become rather saggy with age, so that the woman may end up with a better shaped bosom than her original one. The prosthesis he now uses is made of a silicone gel which moves naturally like the human breast. It doesn't feel quite the same – slightly inert and cold to the touch – but the women I have spoken to look on this as a very minor disadvantage, as I think I might in the same circumstances.

Generally speaking, he prefers to do the implant at the time of the original mastectomy, thus avoiding the trauma of two operations, but this is not always possible. Providing that the woman is in good health and that her skin is elastic and not too tight around the site of the scar, the operation is feasible, two, three or more years later.

It is interesting to note that in spite of the criticism he gets from some doctors, many others are sending him those of their patients whom they regard as suitable and who are very keen to have this cosmetic improvement. I saw one such woman the day after her operation and her obvious delight, which he of course has seen repeated several hundred times, can only be a source of gratification and pleasure to him. Doctors are, after all, human too and in a profession where they see so much unhappiness and suffering about which they can do very little, it seems hard that they should be denied the occasional reward of gratitude for transforming an individual's life. Occasionally and only where it is surgically acceptable, he will do an implant for a woman who does not have a good prognosis, on the grounds that if her mutilation means so much to her, then it is better that she should live with a restored breast even if that life cannot last very long.

I have described this particular doctor's work in this area of cosmetic surgery at some length because he is undoubtedly the leading exponent of it and, as such, deserves credit for his determination in the face of considerable disapproval from some of his colleagues. However, it is also interesting to observe that there are many other surgeons who are now offering implants to their patients at several centres throughout the country. One surgeon told me that he is now doing an average of thirty a week and he is by no means unique. In years to come, this method of conserving the breast is likely to become a routine procedure in breast cancer surgery for many more women.

This is the most exciting and hopeful recent development in breast cancer surgery which gives new hope to women and should encourage more of them to come earlier for treatment. It must surely also be a marvellous new step for surgeons who have become increasingly depressed over the years by the negative results of negative surgery.

However, there is one extension of it which I doubt will ever really catch on in this country, although it has some enthusiastic supporters in the United States. There, many doctors believe that a woman who is known to run a very high risk of developing breast cancer, because, for instance, she has a strong family history of it, should be offered, as a matter of course, a prophylactic bi-lateral, subcutaneous mastectomy followed by implants. To put that into plain English such women are advised to have both natural breasts removed and replaced with prostheses in their twenties before they have a chance to develop a cancer which, of course, may never happen. It's a logical point of view, but is it human or wise? I agree with the surgeon whose work has been described in this chapter and who comments on this argument: 'If you take life that way, you might as well jump off the end of Beachy Head as soon as you can walk.'

10 What else can they do?

*Each case requires repeated individual assessment
if the many different possibilities of therapy are
to be used to the best advantage*
(*Radiotherapy*, M. D. Snelling, 1974)

The author of this statement is the Director of the Meyerstein
Institute of Radiotherapy at the Middlesex Hospital in London
and it comes at the beginning of her chapter in a book on the treatment of breast cancer edited by Professor Sir Hedley Atkins,
founder and, until his retirement, head of the breast unit at Guys
Hospital. She makes it in the context of discussing the various
uses of radiotherapy for the treatment of breast cancer but the
philosophy she expresses is one which is now becoming widely
accepted practice among all the leading doctors in this speciality,
whether they be surgeons, radiologists, endocrinologists or physi-
cians. It is a logical development of the view that breast cancer
should be regarded as a systemic disease right from the start of
treatment.

We have seen how surgeons are incorporating this new thinking into their management of individual patients. This chapter
now looks at other ways of treating breast cancer, which are sometimes used together and sometimes applied on their own or in a
consecutive fashion, depending on the type of tumour, the extent
of its spread (if this can be established), and the stage of the disease. For the sake of clarity each will be discussed separately, but
the reader should bear in mind that they are frequently inter-
dependent and certainly, as far as the doctors are concerned, are
always a matter for combined consideration and repeated consultation when deciding how to treat the individual woman.

Radiotherapy

Radiotherapy is the treatment of disease by radiation energy. It is
designed to destroy tumour cells while leaving healthy tissue

relatively unaffected, although there is always some scarring. These days, the type of energy used is most often a high-energy (megavoltage) X-ray beam which, in skilful hands, where the amount and frequency of the dose is carefully monitored, causes the minimum of damage to healthy tissue. Some reaction, however, is normal and must be expected although it is often no worse than a mild case of sunburn. This energy is similar to, but much more powerful than, the low-energy beams produced by X-rays which are done for diagnostic purposes. Radium and cobalt are other radioactive sources of energy which produce continuous radiation, but neither is now used as much in radiotherapy as it was in the past. In the case of radium this is because it very often causes a strong and painful reaction on healthy tissue, particularly the skin. Where cobalt is concerned, sometimes known as the poor man's megavoltage because it is a cheap form of high-energy radiation, its advantages have been superseded by the latest linear accelerator X-ray machines which produce a far more penetrating and therefore effective beam, particularly on breast tissue.

There are almost as many variations in technique as there are radiotherapists to administer the treatment and women who need it. Each woman is different in shape and size and state of health at the time of treatment. Tumours, as we have seen, also vary greatly in type, size and location. Those which are slow-growing are less sensitive to radiation and may therefore require more prolonged or higher dosage. Others which grow more rapidly are usually more effectively treated by radiotherapy alone. In planning his treatment schedule, the radiotherapist has to take all these and more factors into account which he can only do by careful discussion with the surgeon and the radiologist from the moment that the malignancy has been diagnosed. To quote Miss Snelling again: 'Individualisation and strict accuracy are essential but richly repay the care and time of radiotherapist and radiographer.' The *radiotherapist* is the doctor who plans the treatment and the *radiographer* is the person who operates the machine for delivering the radiation. Then there is the *radiologist* – also a doctor – who interprets the X-rays which are taken for diagnostic purposes. In the case of breast cancer these are called mammograms and they may be taken both before and after the operation. It is, therefore, only after considering the radiologist's investigation and diagnosis, as well as the surgeon's opinion, that the radiotherapist can determine the treatment.

After surgery, radiotherapy is the longest established method of treatment for dealing with breast cancer and, until fairly recently, it was always administered with one end in mind, namely to remove all possible lingering vestiges of malignancy, whether in the breast or in the axillary lymph nodes, after mastectomy. In a word, its value was thought to lie in offering the patient a double insurance that her disease had been eradicated.

The usual procedure was to give every woman who had had a mastectomy – almost invariably a radical until about thirty years ago – a course of routine radiotherapy after her operation. Its efficacy only began to be questioned when people began to look more closely at the mortality figures and it became clear that the method of treatment for the primary cancer (when it first appears) seemed to make no difference to ultimate survival. One of the first to point this out was McWhirter, the Edinburgh radiotherapist, who in 1948 published a study comparing patients who had had either a radical or a simple mastectomy but in all cases the operation had been followed by routine radiotherapy. Approximately half his sample were dead after ten years, irrespective of the operation they had had. He concluded that radical operations were unnecessarily drastic and his advice that all patients should have merely a simple mastectomy followed by routine radiotherapy regardless of whether the lymph nodes had been clinically diagnosed as positive became standard practice in Scotland and known as the Edinburgh technique. What he probably did not foresee was the eventual effect that his conclusions would have on his own speciality, because, as a result of his study, there followed a further flurry of trials both to investigate his claim and to reassess the role of radiotherapy itself.

The most notable of these is the Manchester trial which was based on the Christie Hospital in the 1950s and assessed for ten-year results in 1968. Here patients were compared who were all given a radical mastectomy but they were divided post-operatively into two groups. One group received routine radiotherapy, the other did not. Again, the survival figures showed no difference, not just ten years later, but at any time during the period leading up to ten years. In other words, the same number of patients from both groups died from distant spread of the disease at approximately the same times after their operation, a fact which matters when you think of patients as individual human beings and not as numbers. Furthermore, among those that died who had been in the group not receiving radiotherapy one-third of them never suffered the local recurrence of their disease which meant that they were at least spared the unpleasant after-effects sometimes induced by radiotherapy, particularly at that time when techniques were considerably less refined than they are today. Those patients who did get local recurrence were treated immediately for it with 'on demand' radiotherapy which proved as successful in controlling it as for those who were given the routine post-operative procedure. To express the important findings of this trial (which have since been confirmed by many others) in a more positive way, routine post-operative radiotherapy makes no difference to the survival figures (in that trial 45 per cent of patients from both groups were alive after ten years) so there is no point in giving it until there are signs of local recurrence. However, when it is given on a delayed basis, that is to say as and when it is needed, it works effectively.

I have described this trial in some detail because it is responsible for much of today's revised thinking about radiotherapy. It does not mean that radiotherapy has been superseded as a treatment for breast cancer – indeed there are cases as I describe later in this chapter where it can be used alone, without surgery, to give the best results – but it is no longer regarded as the automatic prophylactic (preventive) in all cases of breast cancer, as a back-up to surgery. In human terms this means that women who don't need it can be spared its side-effects, some of which, like skin reaction, swollen arm and depression may occur almost immediately, and others, like tissue damage, may only appear many years later. However, these side-effects are not invariable and much depends on the skill of the individual radiotherapist. The more carefully he or she (many women are in this field of medicine) discusses each patient's needs with the surgeon, the more likely they are to avoid subsequent trouble for that patient.

Although most doctors now appreciate that radiotherapy is not a necessary preventive measure when it is combined with a mastectomy, many still worry that if they do a simple mastectomy without using Professor Forrest's technique for diagnosing certain important nodes in the chest, they can't know whether the disease has spread to nodes either there or in the axilla. If it has, local recurrence is very likely, so, rather than adopt the wait-and-see policy which can be upsetting for the patient if she has (mistakenly) not been taken into her doctor's confidence and suddenly finds her disease coming back two or three years later in the same place, many doctors prefer to avoid the chance of this happening, either by doing a modified radical which means that the lymph nodes under the arm are also removed (whether or not they prove to be positive on histologic analysis) or they do a simple mastectomy, followed by routine radiotherapy, again regardless of the patient's lymph node status which, in this procedure, can only be assessed clinically. The choice of the individual doctor depends very much on his views about radiotherapy. Those who believe that the possible after-effects of radiotherapy should be avoided, if at all possible, will opt for the modified radical where the fact of removing the lymph nodes also cuts out the need for radiotherapy. Others who are less perturbed about radiotherapy but may be more concerned to do as little mutilation as is compatible with effective surgery will opt for the simple. There is little to choose between the two procedures as far as end result is concerned since both will achieve the same thing, namely a good chance that the disease will not recur locally. In the circumstances it is probably wiser to accept your surgeon's decision because he knows which operation he is happier with and that will make it a better operation for you.

However, before looking at some other uses for radiotherapy it is worth noting that there are now some surgeons who prefer always to do a simple mastectomy and never to follow it up with radiotherapy, even if the lymph nodes do feel swollen on clinical examination, because they argue, first, that removing the lymph nodes lowers the patient's resistance to the disease. (Remember they have an immunological function.) It is certainly true that lymph nodes often swell and then disappear for no particular reason so it seems a pity to remove them unnecessarily when they could be useful. Second, they say that logic is on their side, because as it has been proved that radiotherapy does not have an overall preventive effect on the disease, that is, it can't stop metastasis, what on earth is the point of doing it, until you have definite proof that there is malignancy in the nodes and that it is causing local recurrence. The moment it appears, they treat it at once with a short sharp and effective blast of radiotherapy.

Another important trial (for an account of how clinical trials are organized, read Chapter 11), funded by the Cancer Research Campaign, which includes 2,000 patients and is still in process, is seeking to give definitive answers on this and some of the other questions which still remain about the role of radiotherapy as a first-line treatment for breast cancer. Patients with Stage 1 and Stage 2 disease are randomly divided into two groups, one group getting simple mastectomy alone and the other getting, in addition to the simple mastectomy, the usual routine post-operative radiotherapy. Without going into too much technical detail, the first five-year results indicate, among other things, that although patients with Stage 2 disease do have an increased risk of getting local recurrence, it can still be effectively treated in most cases and doing it on the 'on demand' principle does not hasten the spread of the disease. It also does not appear that routine radiotherapy lowers immunological resistance. Overall there are no differences between either group as far as survival or spread of the disease is concerned. There is little comment a lay person can make when faced with such evidence, but it seems fairly conclusive that while radiotherapy has many uses, it should now never be adopted as an automatic procedure for all patients who have a mastectomy.

Although radiotherapy has now been assigned a less important role for most cases of primary breast cancer there are a few tumours for which it is considered to be the best, sometimes the sole treatment. The fast-growing type has already been mentioned and the reason here is that radiotherapy works quickly to sterilize and halt the growth, whereas there is a very real danger that the surgeon's knife could spread the cancer.

There is also a revived interest in using radiotherapy alone when the tumour is very small (under three centimetres) and there seem to be no enlarged lymph nodes on clinical examination. This operation has much more favour in Europe – France particularly where radiotherapists at the Fondation Curie have, as long ago as the thirties and forties, been doing it on carefully selected patients with, they contend, as good success in survival terms as patients who have had the classical radical mastectomy. In recent years it has also been done on a trial basis in Canada with similarly good results. The leading exponent in that country is Dr Vera Peters who, however, usually precedes the radiotherapy with a wedge excision (lumpectomy). Most doctors in this country are still not very enthusiastic about it, despite the results of the Guys Trial (see page 73) which showed that patients with Stage 1 cancer treated by this method showed as good results, apart from local recurrence, as those who had had a mastectomy.

A Swiss radiologist, Dr P. Veraguth, who is Director of the Department of Radiotherapy at the Inselspital in Berne, also maintains that his results compare extremely well in survival terms providing that certain criteria for selecting suitable patients are strictly observed. In addition to the tumour being small, the breast itself must be small to medium in size because otherwise the radiotherapy will not home in accurately on the tumour. The treatment must be preceded by a mammogram to make sure that there are no other tumours in that breast, or the other one, and the advantages of saving the patient's breast must be weighed up against the possible tissue damage due to the very high dosage needed to make the treatment effective, which may come at a later stage. The breast is likely to become somewhat shrunken and changed in skin texture and sometimes the arm on the same side also becomes rather stiff. Finally, it is essential that the patient always keeps her regular follow-up appointments so that if there is any local recurrence it can be immediately spotted and treated.

Obviously this type of radiotherapy can only be done by doctors who are convinced that it works and know exactly what they are doing because there is an immense skill attached to getting the dose absolutely right, but for those women who fit the criteria, the long-term side-effects may seem negligible compared to the advantage of saving their breast. However, they must be aware of their possibility and it is the duty of the doctor to warn them.

Radiotherapy is also a very effective pain-relieving treatment for cancer which has spread to other parts of the body, the bones in particular. At one time it was thought that irradiation of the breast could cause cancer, but trials have now largely disproved this view, certainly as far as the modern method of giving a high dosage – over a short period to women either before or after an operation – is concerned, and this is also true of the exclusive radiotherapy for small carefully selected tumours which has been described above. Techniques have improved immeasurably in this speciality during the last twenty years, and women who may have known friends or relatives who suffered from acute skin reaction in the past can be reassured that this will not happen to them. Nonetheless, they should be aware that, apart from some physical side-effects which are unavoidable, they may also feel a certain general malaise and depression for a period, which can only partly be ascribed to the unhappiness of having had a mastectomy. Arm lymphoedema also occurs in some women, and ways of coping with this are described in Chapter 13.

Hormone therapy

Ever since a certain Mr Beatson – a surgeon and yet another Scotsman – discovered in 1885 that by removing the ovaries of two of his patients who had advanced breast cancer he was able to halt the disease for a considerable time, doctors have realized that there is undoubtedly a strong relationship between breast cancer and hormones, but what it is exactly, and how best it can be exploited to improve the patient's condition is still, today, not clearly understood.

The basic theory is that many, if not all, breast cancers are hormone-dependent. At the present stage of research it has been established that some of these cancers can be halted, but not permanently cured, either by removing hormone-producing organs like the ovaries or the adrenal glands or suppressing their function with anti-oestrogen agents, or by administering certain hormones – again a paradox which has yet to be explained. The literature on the subject of *hormone* or *endocrine therapy*, to use the medical term, is immense and the views expressed, which are based on innumerable trials, tend to be contrary and confusing, so it is neither useful nor within the scope of this book to review them in any detail. Interested readers who wish to know more are referred to the general bibliography.

This is perhaps the moment to define the differences between the terms 'adjuvant therapy', 'combined modality therapy' and 'symptomatic therapy' all of which are used frequently in the medical literature, but should also be appreciated by women if they want to have a better understanding of the various treatment options. *Adjuvant* means auxiliary or additional and it refers to any treatment such as hormone therapy or chemotherapy which is used at the same time as the primary cancer is first treated in a curative way – that is to say by surgery and possibly radiotherapy as well. *Symptomatic* means what it suggests: this is therapy applied when the cancer gives signs of having reappeared in distant parts of the body. In other words it has definitely become metastatic disease and all four treatments (surgery, radiotherapy, hormone therapy and chemotherapy) can be used, either singly, sequentially, or in various combinations, to control these secondaries. *Combined modality* again means what it suggests: different therapies used in different degrees together, and this type of therapy can be used either at the primary or the secondary stage of the disease. Advanced thinkers like Dr Bernard Fisher in the United States, who is a surgeon and oncologist (cancer specialist) running some of the most promising trials to test chemotherapy, believes that the term 'adjuvant', when applied to hormone and chemotherapy, is misleading for one simple and compelling reason. The logical outcome of accepting that breast cancer is nearly always systemic by the time it is discovered which, as we have seen, is now pretty well proven, is that treatment too should always be systemic. Furthermore, no particular treatment takes precedence over another. Surgery and radiotherapy take care of the local disease: hormone, chemo- and possibly, one day, immuno-therapy, are called upon, as appears appropriate for the individual woman, to treat the disease elsewhere in the body. Therefore, all therapy should be planned on a combined modality approach.

In the case of hormone therapy, it used to be a fairly common procedure to remove a woman's ovaries at the same time as giving her a mastectomy. If she was in the younger age group, this would, of course, give her an artificial menopause and possibly a distressing additional disability to have to endure, but the argument was that since oopherectomy (as this operation is called) was often beneficial in delaying a return of the disease, she might as well have the advantage sooner rather than later. Doctors, today, are far less keen on doing this operation at this early stage because trials have shown that although it certainly can delay the disease coming back, it makes no difference to ultimate survival and it has had an adverse effect on later hormone therapy. Also in many women it makes no difference even to delay, so that is another reason for not putting them through a needless operation. It is interesting that this operation is often called castration, surely a horrible term, made no better by the way one doctor described it to his patient – 'just as easy as spaying your cat and takes no longer' – which suggests that there is more than a little truth in what another doctor told me, namely that it was an operation which was too often done on spec. just because it is so easy. However, there are very good reasons for doing it when the disease has definitely reappeared, especially if the woman is pre-menopausal or not more than five years into her menopause, because if it is successful then, she has the chance of a good remission, relatively free from side-effects and those she does get are obviously preferable to untreated advanced cancer.

Other surgical methods of applying hormone therapy in advanced disease are by removing the adrenal glands (adrenal-ectomy) or the pituitary gland (hypophysectomy). Both are major operations and neither is advisable, unless the doctors are as sure as they can be that they will work. Alternatives to surgery which appear to have much the same effect are irradiation of the ovaries (X-ray treatment) and medically suppressing the adrenals by corticosteroids and other drugs. A much less drastic method in which there is now a great deal of interest because it produces virtually no side-effects is by means of anti-oestrogen drugs which it appears are particularly effective for older women. Several versions are being tried out but Tamoxifen seems to be the most hopeful, especially as it also seems to work for a certain proportion of women who have had Oestrogen Receptor negative tumours (see below). Other trials are going on to see whether a combined treatment of cytotoxic drugs with certain hormones can produce a better result.

Overall, the position of hormone therapy *vis-à-vis* other therapeutic measures is complicated and uncertain. Selection of the right patients at the right moment in their medical condition seems to be the key factor, because when hormone therapy does work for an individual woman it gives her a very good remission. There is a chance now that this careful selection of patients will be made easier by the discovery that at least 70 per cent of breast tumours contain molecules called Oestrogen Receptor protein, the level of which gives a doctor a very good idea of how his patients will respond to hormone therapy. The higher it is the better the chance of a good response. The major problem about this scientific breakthrough is that it is a difficult, time-consuming procedure to test the tumour for this chemical which must be done at the time of removing the tumour and at present can only be done by a few pathologists in a few centres. However, since researchers are hopeful that before long they will find other bio-chemical tumour-markers to assist doctors in their selection of patients, there is a distinct possibility that in the not too remote future, hormone therapy could produce much better results.

Chemotherapy

Over the past twenty years cytotoxic (anti-cancer) drugs have been used to an ever-increasing extent, mainly to treat advanced cancer with the aim of securing good remissions for patients. At first single drugs were used, then, as understanding grew of the way they worked on the tumour and on the body generally, various combinations were and are being tested, with the two-fold aim of improving response and reducing the side-effects, some of which can be most unpleasant. Administered at this stage of the disease, they don't effect a cure but they do achieve control, for varying periods, in much the same way as diabetes is never cured but it can be controlled by drugs.

Today, however, there is a very hopeful and exciting advance in chemotherapy. Trials are beginning to show that if you give certain combinations of these drugs to patients at the time when they first present with the cancer, after mastectomy (and sometimes beforehand as well) there is a chance that you may prevent the disease returning. Results and the conclusions to be drawn from them are still very tentative. Much more testing has to be done and patients who are submitted to this regime, which varies from centre to centre, must be watched for many more years before doctors will be able to make any firm pronouncement about their effectiveness.

The basic theory behind *adjuvant chemotherapy*, that is to say cytotoxic drugs administered at the primary stage of the disease, is based on tumour growth and behaviour. Remember what was said in Chapter 5 about the way tumours double, and that most of this happens before the tumour can be felt or even seen on a mammogram. It is also known that the bigger the tumour becomes the slower its growth, mainly because it doesn't have enough blood supply to feed the extra cells and this also makes it less responsive to chemotherapy. It also happens at some stage during this early growth that certain cancer cells are shed into the blood stream to settle in distant parts of the body. Although there is still a great deal of uncertainty about the exact relationship of these seeded cells to the primary tumour, there is apparently considerable evidence to suggest that when the primary tumour is removed from the breast any such micrometastases (minute spreads) which might otherwise have lain dormant are stimulated into growth. Therefore, goes the argument for chemotherapy, if you can administer the right dose at this stage when these residual cells are very responsive to drugs, just because they are growing, you may be able to knock them all off before they have a chance to develop. If this proves to be true and the right drugs can be found, then this could be the breakthrough that everyone has been looking for, to revolutionize the treatment of breast cancer and offer a much improved chance of cure to many more women.

However, many bridges have to be crossed before that day is reached. Trials are in progress all over the world but the most interesting are those run comparatively by Dr Bernard Fisher in America and Dr Gianni Bonadonna in Milan. Using different drugs (in America it is L-PAM (L-phenylaline mustard) on its own or with another called 5-FU and in Italy it is a combination of three called CMF (cyclophosphamide methotrexate and fluorouracil)), they are giving them to women who have had radical mastectomies and who proved to have positive axillary nodes. Dr Bonadonna published his first results in 1976 after twenty-seven months and he was able to demonstrate a very significant difference between his study group (those who got the drug) and his control group (those who didn't). Only 5.3 per cent of his study patients relapsed with recurrent disease in that time, whereas 24 per cent of the women in the control group relapsed. He was also able to show that whereas the number of nodes which are positive at the time of operation do have a significant bearing on prognosis – the fewer there are the better the outlook – his treatment was equally effective for pre- and post-menopausal women (in other chemotherapeutic regimes pre-menopausal women always seem to do much better than older women).

He has been criticized for leaping into print so early in the trial, mainly because the long-term effects of this drug must be included in any criteria of what constitutes a successful cure. For instance, does this therapy merely delay the return of the disease or does it actually improve survival? Just over two years is after all a very brief span in a possible period of up to twenty years. Is there any danger that it could ultimately cause cancer?

Bonadonna, whose name translated means Good Woman – very apt if he does prove ultimately to have found a new curative treatment for breast cancer – is very careful himself to stress that these are only preliminary findings and that much work has yet to be done. However, many responsible doctors who personally wish him well, fear that his premature publication will encourage other less skilled and over-enthusiastic doctors to rush into prescribing CMF or other combinations of drugs without selecting their patients carefully enough and without doing the proper follow-up studies which would make their treatment worthy of comparison with properly controlled and evaluated trials. It is more than a worry; it is a fact that many patients, more in America than here, are being prescribed chemotherapy injudiciously and to no avail because it is not suitable for their condition or their type of disease. In an area of medicine where *no one*, as yet, knows the final answers and *no one* has found the wonder drug, the qualities of open-mindedness combined with extreme caution, plus a fair dose of humility are essential.

The major problem about all anti-cancer drugs is that they are extremely toxic and patients on a regimen must be watched very carefully to ensure that the misery induced by their side-effects, which can sometimes be very severe, doesn't outweigh any benefits they may confer. Doctors are increasingly concerned about the quality of life their treatments offer to women. We have seen that there are distinct disadvantages in this respect with surgery, radiotherapy and hormone therapy. Even more so is this true with chemotherapy where side-effects include alopecia (baldness), extreme nausea, cystitis, diarrhoea and numbness in the finger tips which make it difficult for a woman to do the simplest household and personal tasks. They all disappear immediately the drugs are stopped – hair grows back, for instance, as strongly as before and a wig is worn in the interval – but when the treatment may continue for as long as a year, the individual woman suffering the side-effects may wonder despairingly whether it is worthwhile. This is especially true with adjuvant chemotherapy, because normally a woman feels physically well after a mastectomy especially if she has not had radiotherapy, but she may have emotional and psychological problems to contend with, which can be severely aggravated by aggressive chemotherapy.

On the other hand, unless the trials are made, on as large and rapid a scale as possible, the final answers won't be forthcoming for years and if they prove to be as good as the interim results suggest they may be, then that delay could mean that the next generation of women will be denied their life-saving benefit. But if today's women are to suffer in the cause of tomorrow's cure, then they must at least be granted the right to know why they are being prescribed the drug. In the case of recurrent disease, the advantages of chemotherapy are usually more obvious – a remission is an improvement on illness – but the woman who is prescribed chemotherapy immediately after mastectomy should ask her doctor for the reason. If he responds that she is in a trial and explains the treatment, and the side-effects she must expect, then she can be reassured and accept the regimen in the confidence that she will be getting optimum medical care.

Immunotherapy

In the last seventy years there have been many attempts to treat breast and other forms of cancer by immunotherapy, but the results have always been disappointing. Strictly speaking, since it is still so experimental, it has no right to be included in a chapter such as this which describes valid and long-established methods of treatment. However, it is potentially a very promising area of research, not only for itself as an eventual form of treatment, but also for the light that increasing knowledge about the body's defence mechanisms against malignant disease throws on all the existing treatments.

For example, the fact that surgery, by whatever method, doesn't have any effect on the long-term outcome, but it does cause a marked improvement on the immediate condition of most patients with breast cancer, suggests two possibilities: either that removing the breast tumour reduces the rate of spread in other organs, or that once the body no longer has to fight the primary tumour it can better summon its defences to cope with all the scattered cancer cells. On the other hand, if the theory described on page 93 is correct, which suggests that these same tiny growths immediately become more active when the primary tumour is removed, then the host defences (medical term for body in this context) may still not be able to cope.

Since this theory supplies the basic rationale for adjuvant chemotherapy, a new problem arises because many of the cyto-toxic drugs used in this therapy are known to be strongly im-munosuppressive, that is to say, they weaken or even totally neutralize the body's own defence mechanisms. Studies show that chemotherapy is always more successful in cases where the drugs do not have this dangerously lowering effect on the patient's immunological defences, but at the moment the only known way to counteract it is by very carefully monitoring the size, number and frequency of drug doses. Here is yet another strong argu-ment for saying that doctors who prescribe chemotherapy should do so under strictly observed trial conditions because, in the hands of people who don't fully understand their potency, these drugs can do more harm than good.

A different sort of monitoring problem occurs when deciding how to check a patient for her level of immunological com-petence, that is to say, judging how capable her body is of fighting malignancy before, during and after therapy. The testing methods now in use tend to be cumbersome and unreliable, yet it is vital that this aspect of immunological research be refined because this knowledge is necessary if the medical team is to make a fully in-formed decision about the type of treatment to give to an individ-ual patient.

In the case of radiotherapy, there is much more positive evi-dence, coming, among other things, from trials described earlier in this chapter, to show that destroying the lymph nodes by a routine course of post-operative radiotherapy, especially where they are not affected by the cancer, could definitely be unwise for the patient's long-term wellbeing. How the lymph nodes and other defence mechanisms in the body do their work is still very imprecisely understood; indeed, like every other area of immuno-logical research it's easier to define the many gaps rather than the few hard facts. However, one fact which does emerge from both clinical and experimental evidence is that regional lymph nodes (those in close proximity to a tumour) will respond immunologically, that is to say, fight the tumour, at least for a while, presumably until they are overcome by its growing strength and size.

Bearing this in mind and remembering, too, that cancer is probably always in the body system by the time it is diagnosed, it is now becoming an accepted principle underlying any type of treatment for breast cancer that great care should be taken, wherever possible, not to destroy the body's defence mechanisms needlessly. Hence a reason for conservative surgery – to avoid doing too much damage to local tissue; similarly with radiotherapy – only to be done when it is the best method for a particular cancer or to treat a local recurrence but not as a matter of course. With chemotherapy the treatment is systemic and correspondingly great care is required because the harm that could be caused by injudiciously reducing the body's defences is more widespread and more insidious.

Immunology has a long way to go and much remains to be revealed before it can be regarded as a useful therapeutic arm of medicine, but even at its present embryonic stage it sounds a suitably cautious note for those who, in their enthusiasm for man-made remedies, forget that Nature too has a vital role to play in the curing and healing process; furthermore, to ignore or flout her is to invite disaster.

11 Informed consent

Throughout this book I refer to clinical trials, comparing various methods of treatment for breast cancer, which have been done and are carried out in ever-increasing numbers all over the world. The ones I have specifically mentioned are a tiny fraction of the whole, and to enumerate them in any detail would be irrelevant to the purpose of this book which is to present an overall view of breast cancer in lay language, but any reader who does wish to know more about them and the conclusions which have been drawn from them will find references to all the major ones in one or other of the books listed in the general bibliography on page 156.

Controlled clinical trials are very important both for the doctors who are re-evaluating their approach to breast cancer and looking at new ways of managing it on the combined modality model, and for any woman who now, or in the future, is under threat of getting this disease. However, the results which emerge from any trial are only valid and useful if the trial itself has been conducted according to a strict protocol. This means that it has a clearly defined objective and it must be planned in accordance with certain rules and criteria which every participating doctor understands, accepts and conscientiously adheres to.

The purpose of most controlled trials is to find out which of two methods of treatment is more effective. In the case of cancer, this could mean comparing a new drug with an established one, or with no drug; one type of surgical procedure with another; radiotherapy in conjunction with surgery, or on its own; a certain method of hormone therapy against a certain method of chemotherapy. The permutations are infinite, but the procedures for applying them are fairly simple and rigorous. The investigators must know what questions they want answers to and they must be worth asking; therefore, it is better to confine themselves to a comparison of two treatments which are different enough from each other to make the result significant, but that result can only be positive or null. What it cannot be is strongly negative in the sense that the new treatment as a result of comparison with a standard method proves to be distinctly worse, either as far as delaying death or improving the quality of life is concerned. This is very relevant where a new drug is being tested, so before it comes to the point of being used in a large-scale clinical trial, it must have gone through very exhaustive tests to check for side-effects and other undesirable features, first with animals and then with patients who have advanced incurable disease on whom no other therapy has any effect. These patients must be told that they are being given a new drug and their consent must be obtained beforehand. Only then and only if the effects look promising, can this drug be tried on a slightly larger group of patients who also have advanced disease but for whom an alternative therapy is still possible. Again their consent must be obtained. If the drug passes all these tests and still looks good, then it can be tried out in a controlled clinical trial on a much larger number of patients who have been selected according to certain criteria. For instance, they may all have received the same initial treatment for a stage two cancer and they may all fall within a certain age group. This is particularly important in breast cancer where it is known that the disease is biologically different in pre- and post-menopausal women. (What causes that difference is still not precisely known but it is likely to be connected with varying levels of hormonal activity.) This selected group of patients is then randomly allocated to one or other of the treatments. Random means exactly that. Neither the doctors conducting the trial nor those who have agreed to participate in it by putting forward those of their patients who fit the selection criteria can know in advance which patient is getting which treatment. Furthermore, they must be entirely agnostic about both forms of treatment because if a doctor thinks that one treatment is definitely superior to the other, he clearly has no right to submit his patients to the possibility of not getting it. Finally he has the undisputed right to withdraw any patient from the trial if he feels that the treatment prescribed is proving unsuitable for that individual.

The ethical implications of such trials are profound and should be as well understood by the patient as by the doctor. The doctor's role is clear. He can only participate if he is genuinely unbiased and totally committed to obeying all the instructions contained in the protocol which will include initial treatment and follow-up. The patient's role is not always so clearly spelled out, yet the concept of 'informed consent' is something which exercises all conscientious doctors. Their dilemma is obvious. How are they going to say to their patients – 'Look, there are these two treatments and frankly we don't know which one is better, so on the toss of a coin you will receive one or the other,' without running the risk of losing the vital trust and confidence of their patients. The problem becomes even knottier when the alternative treatment is no treatment at all.

To take a simple example: there is more than one trial going on at the moment to compare the advantages of a simple mastectomy followed by immediate radiotherapy against a simple mastectomy followed by a watch policy which means that the woman only gets radiotherapy at a later date if she has local recurrence, that is to say the cancer reappears on or near the site of the original tumour. In some ways this is a comparatively easy trial to justify and to explain to the patient at the outset because other trials have clearly demonstrated that radiotherapy makes no difference to the overall cure rate, but it does have a markedly good effect on controlling local disease. Therefore the doctor can say in total honesty to the patient who has been randomly picked for mastectomy without radiotherapy that her prognosis is good, she doesn't need radiotherapy at this stage but if she does she will get it at once and the trouble will be cleared up immediately. However, what she may not be told is that she has a right to refuse this option if she so wishes.

A much more difficult example is when the comparison lies between administering a certain anti-cancer drug to the study group and giving nothing to the control group. Strictly speaking, those who randomly fall into the control group should be told that they are not getting the drug but doctors admit that they find this is very difficult. In America, where patients are much more alert to their rights and much more conditioned to the idea – not always a good one – that some treatment, any treatment, is better than none, these trials can run into considerable difficulties. In this country many doctors tend to duck the issue by allowing their patients a degree of informed consent. What this means is that they will tell those patients who fall into the study group that a new drug is being tried out on them which has been producing some very good results for patients with their particular condition, all of which will be absolutely true and, therefore, in most cases, is likely to be readily accepted by the patient. However, patients coming into the control group may not be told anything, probably not even made aware that they are in a trial. On medical grounds, this can be justified because while it is true to say that they are not getting the new treatment, the benefits of which have yet to be assessed definitively which is why it is on trial, they are getting the standard treatment which is recognized as the best that is currently available and they can be certain that everything possible is being done for them, short of this extra. However, ethically a quibble remains because such patients are being denied the right to give their informed consent.

One way of getting round this problem is to conduct the trial on a 'double blind' basis which means that it is not just the patient who doesn't know whether the pill she is getting is the real thing or a placebo, but the doctor administering it is as much in the dark as herself. Providing that both doctor and patient are aware that the trial is going on and that the patient knows that she has an equal random chance of being allocated to either group, this is probably acceptable, but some doctors worry about this too because they fear that if a patient knows that she may well be getting only a placebo, this in itself will influence her personal recovery and, therefore, the outcome of the trial. It is after all an understandable and quite normal reaction to underrate everything connected with your treatment if you suspect that part of it may not be genuine.

There is another way of surmounting these problems. Instead

of doing a randomized trial, treatments can be compared historically. This way the investigators look at the survival figures for a large number of patients over a period of years who have had a certain treatment and then compare equal numbers of similar patients now receiving a different treatment. The difficulty with this type of trial is that you can never be certain that you are looking at two precisely matched groups of patients. Minor variations in the way patients have been selected for a particular treatment or in the way that that treatment has been administered in the past may not be apparent when the comparison is being made, but may in fact have a pronounced and distorting effect on the conclusions which are finally drawn.

There are several significant factors in analysing trials. Time and the numbers of patients involved are probably paramount. If you are trying out a new method you want to know as quickly as possible whether it is producing better survival rates, so it follows that a very long-term trial defeats its own end because it is likely that both investigators and patients will all be dead before it is concluded. It may be overtaken by other trials against which it will also be matched. Numbers matter because if you have enough patients in the trial, small problems can be picked up early, modifications made without altering the basic outline of the protocol or the treatment can be halted outright if it is seen to be counter-productive. Also important is the quality of life that the new treatment offers. Misery for individual patients who have been put on to a given regimen can never be justified in the cause of establishing a scientific fact. This final point is a strong argument in favour of controlled trials because if there is any such danger, as for instance with administering anti-cancer drugs, some of which are extremely toxic and can be most distressing in their effect, it is most unwise to subject patients to such treatment until it has been critically assessed in a trial and proven to have long-term advantages which outweigh the immediate disadvantages.

Another very strong argument in favour of controlled clinical trials is that the standard of care which every patient receives, irrespective of which group she is assigned to, is likely to be of a much better quality than she might get in routine practice. This is because the participating doctors must conform to the strict rules of the protocol which not only define the treatment but demand very careful and persistent follow-up. It is obviously quite useless for the purposes of assessment to treat large numbers of patients if you then lose them afterwards, and follow-up, as we have seen earlier, is an important element of the continuing care which all women who have had breast cancer must have.

All in all, controlled clinical trials for breast cancer are valuable and necessary, but to be truly effective and ultimately beneficial, coordination and control are the key words. The task of the recently established Breast Trials Coordinating Committee in this country is to assist with the former. This Committee which is widely representative of all the specialities in the treatment of breast cancer acts primarily as an information bank. Doctors who are keen to set up a clinical trial can find out whether their efforts are being duplicated elsewhere; they can seek advice on how to draw up a protocol or, on the basis of the information they receive, they may decide that they will get better results by joining forces with another group planning a similar trial. They can also be kept abreast of the latest developments in cancer research. At the moment, there are far too many small trials going on which cost a lot of money and a lot of effort but will be ultimately valueless because they will never be able to achieve the numbers which are essential for a statistically sound result.

Many doctors are particularly concerned about the current enthusiasm for giving chemotherapy to patients with early cancer, a practice which is widespread in America and beginning to catch on here in certain quarters, because they feel that the results have not yet been submitted to sufficient testing to justify the physical and mental distress which such a regimen invariably causes. This is why control is so necessary but it can only be exerted if the grant-giving bodies such as the Medical Research Council, the Cancer Research Campaign, the Imperial Cancer Research Fund and Tenovus, to name four of the leading organizations, are also kept fully informed. Many of the research projects are of course devised and funded by themselves, but many others are organized by outside groups. Nobody wants to dampen the enthusiasm of a group of doctors who believe that they have an important and interesting question to ask about a certain treatment, but at the same time, the innate conservatism of the British medical profession here works to the patient's advantage rather than otherwise. Just as in surgery the majority of British doctors have advanced by doing more conservative, that is to say, fewer radical mutilating operations, so in the new and potentially very fruitful field of chemotherapy, the majority prefer to proceed cautiously.

Where I think they have sometimes been less commendable is in their lack of candour towards patients participating in a clinical trial, and it is for this reason that I have explained the function and procedures of such trials in some detail. There will always be some people who will not want to know anything about their treatment and that deliberately chosen ignorance may be their way of coping with their illness. As such it should be respected and unwelcome information should not be forced upon them, but when a patient does want to know, then she has a right to honest answers. This is undoubtedly an extra burden for the doctor but as we shall see in Part Three there are ways of sharing this burden and in helping the patient to understand and accept what is happening the doctor helps himself. If 'informed consent' is to mean anything at all, then the first essential must be that the patient knows that she has this right and the second that she understands what it entitles her to, which is: unambiguous information about why she has been selected for a certain trial; what the reasons for it are; and what the doctors hope to achieve by it.

Having stated all this and without wishing to sound a paradox I believe that the patient who is allowed to exercise her right to informed consent is also more likely to accept her treatment, because she now understands the reasons for it. Her confidence in her doctor is also more likely to be reinforced by his frank response to her inquiries. She cannot expect to comprehend all the medical reasons behind the choice of a particular treatment, because she doesn't have the expertise or knowledge, but she will be assured that her individual welfare is his prime concern, which of course it is.

part three

The whole woman

12 Your mind

Breast cancer attacks your body. Mastectomy is, and will continue for some time yet, to be the first and best method of counter-attack. This means that most women who have breast cancer must also face living with a lasting reminder of that assault on their body and, inevitably, this harsh truth will afflict their mind and spirit as well. Probably no woman who has had a mastectomy escapes suffering some measure of psychological and emotional damage. In some cases this may be very severe. As with the physical disease, if the injuries inflicted on the psyche are not recognized by her doctors, or are kept secret by the woman herself, then there is no chance of healing them, and to those who suffer them the mental scars left by a profound psychological disturbance can be more real and terrible than their physical counterpart.

The woman who has had a mastectomy needs mental rehabilitation as much as she needs advice and sympathetic understanding about her physical problems. This is why I have put the mind before the body in this section because it is her mental attitudes which will condition her physical responses. Any woman in this situation needs all the help she can get to help her help herself back to a full and complete recovery. A positive outlook is essential if she is to resume her normal social, family and working life as quickly as possible.

It may seem surprising to be so insistent on this point, but it is a sad fact that only very recently have some members of the medical profession begun to recognize this truth. Far too many doctors still refuse to regard it as any of their business how their patients feel before or after they have performed their operation. To some degree this is explained by the surgeon's typical view of disease which is that he cures it with the knife. He cuts the tumour out, *ipso facto* the source of trouble has been removed and with that act he believes that he has fulfilled his responsibility towards his patient. Partly, it is because he fears his own emotions if he allows himself to become too involved with the emotional problems of his patients. He may well sense that they exist, indeed he would have to be grossly insensitive if he did not, but he is uncertain how to cope with them, therefore he ignores them.

'They're frightened to tell you anything because they're afraid you're going to freak out on them,' one woman told me bitterly, and then added: 'You get more silence than anything. If you don't ask they tell you nothing.' Perhaps she was particularly unfortunate in her hospital. The fact that they even omitted to make an appointment for her follow-up and when she did finally telephone some months later was met with the blithe response, oh dear me, yes, they had forgotten all about her, suggests that she was, but her experience in varying degrees of callousness has been repeated to me over and over again. Even those women who were most enthusiastic and confident about the medical care they had received usually remembered some incident when they had been met by an offhand or dismissive manner. Often they would excuse the doctor or nurse in question by saying that they realized how busy they were and that they couldn't be expected to deal with every little moan, or answer every question.

But can't they? Should it not be an integral part of good medical management that the patient's inquiries and natural anxieties are dealt with as carefully as the physical symptoms are treated? To show that I have not picked these complaints out of the air, let me now quote a surgeon who has completely reorganized his breast clinic since he realized how much mental anguish the traditional aloof attitudes were causing.

'When I first came,' he said, 'we did it very badly. We all walked into the room with a great retinue behind and said, "You've got breast cancer. You've got to have your breast off." Perhaps not quite as badly as that but almost. Of course, we never saw what happened afterwards. The patients said nothing, but after we'd gone they would break down and cry in Sister's arms.' Now he has a nurse with long experience and skill who is part of the team, talks to the women beforehand and tells them what to expect at the examination. Upsetting information is broken gently and the nurse who stays with them afterwards becomes a familiar friend and someone to confide in because she also attends the mastectomy clinic. This practice is still far too rare, but I noticed that wherever something along these lines was being done for patients, the consultant was always keen to introduce me to his nurses, praising their skill and the help they gave him with any patient who was particularly upset. Such attitudes make a refreshing change from the usual authoritarian stance where patients are required to conform to the strictly observed hierarchical structure with doctors remote and distant, way up at the top, nurses, radiographers and other lesser mortals bustling and scurrying to obey their bidding and the patient finds herself pushed right down to the bottom of the heap. The object she may be, of their combined battery of skills and attention, but the woman who fears she has cancer wants to feel she is more than a body exhibiting an interesting symptom. This is a moment in her life when she feels deeply threatened. Her femininity, her relationships, even her life may be at stake. She wants to feel she is still a person, a woman; certainly not the mere object of detached scientific curiosity.

Proper communication between doctor and patient and between patient and all the other hospital staff with whom she may later come into contact is very important at every stage of treatment. Chapter 4 looked at the ways GPs can sometimes misunderstand their patients or refuse to take them seriously even to the extent of dangerously delaying referral to a consultant. Two very interesting pieces of research, one done at a London hospital and the other in Oxford, revealed that communication leaves much to be desired all along the line. The GP may be very vague about the treatment his patient can expect if the lump turns out to be malignant or frighten her by his excessively gloomy reaction when he confirms that she needs further investigation.

When she does get to the hospital, the doctor may be cruelly blunt in the manner described earlier or be unconvincingly bland, using phrases like, 'you've got nothing to worry about', which seldom fool her. Even when she gives him verbal cues with remarks like, 'I've been on nerve pills 'or 'I've been out of my mind with worry' he may ignore them, whether deliberately or because he is insensitive is difficult to establish, but the effect is far from reassuring. Evasive behaviour like this makes the patient increasingly concerned and convinced that the doctor is holding back something sinister. This is a bad start to her programme of treatment and it becomes worse if he continues to deflect her questions after she knows that she will probably have to lose her breast. Signing the consent form which often means that she agrees to a mastectomy if the frozen section proves to be malignant can be a particularly harrowing moment and must be handled carefully, not as happened to one woman. 'The form was just pushed under my nose with the doctor saying "sign there" and it wasn't until I read it that I realized I had breast cancer. When I asked him, was it true? he just said "You've got nothing to worry about." No explanation, nothing.'

After a mastectomy it continues to be very important for the doctor to be as honest and straightforward with the patient as possible without confusing her with a mass of scientific information which she may not understand. Euphemisms like 'we caught it on the turn' or 'we caught it in time before it became cancer' fool no one, least of all the woman who knows that you don't lose a breast lightly. There are of course many thousands of women every year who have mastectomies for severe benign disease, but in every case those women know that they don't have cancer. Women who do have cancer have an equal right to know the truth.

To quote Dr Peter Maguire, a psychiatrist who has done a great deal of research into the psychological effects of having a mastectomy, those women who are denied the truth or given roundabout answers or even conflicting information by different members of the staff, end up by believing no one and nothing. 'Fear of being lied to understandably made them angry, suspicious, and disinclined to believe the truth if or when it was finally offered.' Often the lying is quite unnecessary and very disturbing to the sensitive patient, but even when the information is serious, doctors should always think carefully before they withhold it. For instance, the woman who has not had an operation because her cancer was too advanced may be told that 'it was not cancer but could turn into it unless treated with radiotherapy'. This is appalling for the woman concerned who inevitably is going to realize sooner or later that she has not been told the truth. Her confidence in her treatment and her doctor will be destroyed at a time when she needs as much support and understanding as she can get and it surely cannot help the doctor in his task of persuading his patient that he is doing his best for her.

This is an extreme situation and I don't wish to belittle the enormous difficulties, especially of communication, that doctors treating cancer patients have to face every day of their lives, but if this is their area of specialization, then they must accept that creating an honest relationship with their patients is fundamental to their treatment. Of course not every patient wants to be told the facts. Many will say something like, 'Don't tell me the details. I know you're doing the best you can. I leave it to you,' and if that is how an individual wants to cope with her illness, then her wishes should be respected. But most women want to know what is wrong with them, even if they are afraid to ask directly. A doctor should be tuned in to unspoken questions and be ready to spend a little time finding out what each of his patients feels about her illness and how much she knows or suspects already. By talking and listening to her, he will then be able to gauge how much information she really wants. Experience is all-important and the more he does this the better he will become at imparting it in the proportion and manner that is right for the individual woman.

Another interesting fact which comes out of Dr Maguire's research is that although doctors often claim that they do precisely this, tailoring their communications to the different needs and temperaments of their patients, in practice few of them do. They tend to inflexibility and to rely on well-worn phrases like the ones quoted earlier. I am sure that most of the doctors I spoke to were honourable exceptions to this rule. Many of them made a special point of explaining to me exactly how they tell their patients that they have cancer and why they are having a particular treatment, confirming Dr Maguire's finding that this is a strategy which pays dividends because 'the women felt the surgeon understood their attitudes to their illness, while the surgeons knew exactly what the anxieties were that they needed to counter.'

From the moment a woman discovers a lump in her breast to the time when she wakes up after her operation to find that her worst fears have been confirmed, she will be living in hell. There is no lesser way of describing her state of mind throughout this period, whoever she is and no matter whether she be young or old, married or single. Fear of death, which is immediately suggested by the dread word cancer, is usually uppermost in her thoughts, closely followed by the dread of mutilation and pain and all the implications that that carries for her in her personal life. Many women, when warned that they must expect a mastectomy, react with the words, 'How can I tell my husband?' They fear his rejection and that he will be repelled by a wife without a breast. Mothers are seized with dread that they may never live to see their children grow up. Single women fear that they will never again have a lover. Elderly women who may already have suffered the loss of their husband cannot imagine how they can survive this new blow on their own. Lonely women will feel utterly bereft and friendless. Even the woman who is lucky to be surrounded by a loving family and friends may now feel terribly alone and unwilling to confide in those who are closest to her, because she feels she can't endure the pain and unhappiness they will be feeling for her.

She experiences mounting tension and stress as she goes through the diagnostic procedures, which will be heightened if hospital staff appear indifferent to her feelings or too busy to talk to her. However, if she can find someone to confide in at this stage, either a nurse or a friend or a stranger who has been introduced to her because she has been through the same experience, she will immediately feel some relief. Some women said that their anxiety lessened from the moment they entered hospital and knew that the decision had, in a sense, been taken out of their hands.

'It was such a relief to be tucked up in bed and know that I was being cared for by people who knew what they were doing.' Another woman described it as 'like waiting for the war to start. It's more frightening beforehand but once you've had cancer it's not nearly as bad. You feel you know what you are fighting and that you can do something about it.' Another was sustained by the words of a friend who had also had a mastectomy and wished her 'good luck with your adventure'.

After a mastectomy, women's immediate reactions vary quite considerably, depending to some extent on their own personal characters and the way they think of themselves in relation to their bodies, but much also depends on how they have been prepared, both for the possibility of mastectomy and the after-effects they should expect. Sometimes they are not told quite simple physical facts such as that it is normal to feel numbness followed by a sensation of constriction and possibly some pain but that this can be quickly alleviated and doesn't last. They may not know what kind of operation they have had or become very worried because the woman in the next bed is getting different treatment. They may be frightened by the tubes which are put in for a few days to drain the wound.

If the doctor has been over-reassuring beforehand that he is certain that the lump will prove to be harmless, a woman will feel she has been deceived and she may react bitterly, angrily, or withdraw into silent depression. Many women have told me that despite their doctor's misplaced optimism, they always felt that it would turn out to be malignant, but waking to find this fear confirmed didn't help them to accept it.

Hospital staff who refuse to recognize these absolutely natural reactions by maintaining a breezy cheerful manner or alternatively taking it personally when the patient's distress spills out in complaints only intensify her misery. Here again it is essential that her questions should be answered frankly and not in the unnerving manner described by one woman whose surgeon always avoided direct contact with her. Instead he would stand a distance away from her bed 'muttering' to the sister, while glancing from time to time in her direction. 'What they don't realize,' she said 'is that it's not what you know which upsets you but what you don't know.' A simple, obvious truth, one would have thought, yet too often disregarded.

Occasionally, women are overwhelmed by quite a different reaction, almost a euphoria that they have been touched by death and emerged alive. One woman describes the whole experience as 'a spiritual adventure' which is still going on many years later. She said that after the operation she felt happier than she had done for a long time. Life seemed enormously sweet and the whole world very beautiful and she was immensely glad to be alive in it. She was asked to talk to the nurses five days after her mastectomy and says that she gave them a manic lecture about how wonderful it was and how marvellous she felt. Six months later a depression set in which took a year to lift.

Few women can escape a period when they will feel very low and negative about themselves as women. Losing a breast is a form of bereavement and if they are to work through it success- fully they must be allowed to grieve. If a woman has always in- vested a great deal in her bodily appearance, and particularly in her bosom, or if she feels that her husband will mind enormously about her different shape, then those feelings are likely to be intensified and progressively worsen unless she is given some very positive help and encouragement. Practical action to restore her to physical health and look the way she was before her operation is described in the next chapter.

Here I am going to describe the psychological support system which a few, far too few, hospitals are just beginning to set up for their mastectomy patients. I have dwelt at some length on the things that can and do go wrong because I believe it is vital that hospital staff review now their whole approach to the severe emotional stress that women in this situation undoubtedly suffer and which, so often, is aggravated rather than relieved by the unthinking behaviour and attitudes of people who have not been trained to understand the problem. If the word gets around that something can be done which doesn't cost too much money, then perhaps more hospitals will be encouraged to set up something similar for their patients.

The Royal Marsden Hospitals in London and Sutton have

each appointed a clinical nurse consultant who has been trained in counselling and fitting prostheses (breast forms) over and above having the normal nursing qualifications. She has special responsibility for mastectomy patients whom she meets for the first time when they come to the outpatient clinic for their initial examination. At this stage, they don't, of course, know their diagnosis, but they will be very worried and she can allay some of their fears by describing the diagnostic procedure and listening to their problems.

For instance, if a woman can be told something quite simple like the order of events and the time schedule she can expect if she is to be called into hospital, this will enable her to start making arrangements for her family or about her job. Then, when she does come in for the operation, she is met by a familiar person who will spend as much time with her as she wants before the operation, telling her what it involves and what she will feel like when she comes round from the anaesthetic. She will also try and meet the husband or whoever is the close relative or companion if she has not already done so at the first outpatient visit because it is vital to establish this link as early as possible.

Husbands are especially important figures in their wives' recovery but they often need special counselling too. Fortunately few of them reject their wives in the way that the women so often fear, but they too are frightened of what this is going to do to their marriage, and nervous about how to make the first approaches, especially if the woman herself has become very withdrawn and rejecting. Sometimes they do what the nurse described to me as 'an ostrich act', refusing to discuss anything because they are afraid of saying the wrong thing which can backfire disastrously on their wife who then imagines that she was right after all. She has been rejected. So the nurse can do a lot in this area to clear up misunderstandings and help the couple face the problem together.

Other women don't want to tell anyone, not even their families, about what is happening to them, some going so far as to pretend that they are going into hospital for some other quite minor operation. Who women tell is their own business and everyone should be allowed to make their own decision about this, but in such cases the role of the clinical nurse consultant (or liaison nurse as she is called in Dr Maguire's hospital where a similar system operates) may be even more important to the woman. She must have someone to talk to and who better than a calm, sympathetic, knowledgeable outsider?

The nurse appears at the bedside soon after the patient has come round from her operation and although she doesn't do any nursing herself – in fact, she has to be very careful not to step on the toes of the ward sister who might naturally resent this as a usurpation of her authority – she closely follows the patient's recovery. She discusses prostheses and bras with her, shows her models and gives her a lightly fitting prosthesis which she will wear for the first few weeks. She discusses the patient's exercises with her and any problems she may have, either in hospital or that she fears are waiting for her at home. She acts as a friend, a guide and a counsellor and when the patient goes home, she continues to be available to her, on the telephone or to make a home visit, if she is asked, or if she thinks it is necessary. She also runs a non-medical mastectomy clinic where she sees the patient at regular follow-up intervals, and in addition to checking that she is happy with her prosthesis she can discuss other problems with her as well. She is offering total nursing care.

The clinical nurse consultant I talked to was totally absorbed by her work. It's very draining mentally but she goes home to her family and switches off completely which is a good thing, because although she must be involved with her patients she cannot allow herself to be completely taken over by them and their problems. She also has to tread a very delicate path between doctors and other nurses on the one side, and on the other, the patient. Interestingly enough, where there is opposition to such a scheme (and it does not exist in these hospitals) it comes less from the doctors than from other nurses who argue that it is an invasion of their caring role.

Both this nurse consultant and Dr Peter Maguire would like to try out other forms of therapy, for instance group sessions for the first few months after the operation where patients who had been treated at the same time could discuss any difficulties and share experiences. The nurse would guide the session so that medical questions could also be answered and possibly other hospital personnel could also be involved, like physiotherapists to do arm exercises, or social workers to deal with anything particularly intractable in the home situation.

Specially trained volunteers are another idea. These would be women who have had a mastectomy themselves and who are willing to counsel new mastectomy patients. This type of aid has become very well established and accepted in America due to the drive and zeal of one woman, Terese Lasser, who created the Reach to Recovery programme after her own mastectomy in 1952 when she was horrified to discover that she could get no help of any sort, not even basic instruction about arm exercises or prostheses.

Something similar here is the admirable Mastectomy Association, founded by Betty Westgate in 1971, but these volunteers have not received any training like, for example, marriage guidance counsellors do, and their object is simply to offer practical advice. (More about both these organizations in the next chapter.)

Sad to say, these imaginative schemes meet with a great deal of scepticism and indeed obduracy from many doctors, some of whom still persist in refusing to recognize that mastectomy patients have a problem at all. Yet there is plenty of evidence in the medical literature if they would only look for it, and there are also some good results coming from America and Canada where this type of counselling, both on a group and individual basis, is much more advanced and widely accepted. Doctors seem to be particularly antagonistic to lay volunteers, suggesting that they will frighten the patients with their own experiences or interfere with their medical treatment by putting subversive ideas into their heads. This attitude is close to paranoia in certain hospitals where even the helpful, medically approved leaflets distributed free by the Mastectomy Association are not allowed.

Over and over again, women complained to me that nobody told them anything, that they wished they had known what to expect, particularly after they got home. Often they were not even instructed in arm exercises. While they are in hospital, they may be lulled into a false sense of security because everything is being done for them, but when they get home suddenly all sorts of problems can hit them, and make it very hard for them to come to terms with their future. Most women will be able to throw away their emotional crutches pretty fast, particularly if they are lucky enough to be able to call on someone like the clinical nurse consultant whose work has been described here. Some, however, are being psychologically crippled for life for lack of elementary understanding and action at a time when the injury can still be healed. And when these women suffer, they are not alone because their unhappiness brings misery into their family and working life. We have seen that there has been a profound change of mind regarding the physical aspects of breast cancer; another such re-evaluation is now needed to accept that breast cancer also has psychological effects which must be countered by professional treatment.

13 Your body

Before you have your operation you will have signed a consent form agreeing to a mastectomy. In those hospitals where the system is to do a biopsy, frozen section and then a mastectomy, should it prove necessary, all at the same time, you may go to sleep, still hoping against hope that you will wake up feeling and looking the same woman that you were before your nightmare started. Where, however, the diagnosis is done in two stages or where the carcinoma is so obvious to the surgeon's trained eye, and he has told you so, you will know as you sign it that there is no going back. By putting your name to that form you have agreed to lose a precious part of yourself.

An abstract consent is different from the concrete reality. Even in those hospitals where all that can be done is done before-hand by doctors and nurses to inform and prepare the patient by sympathetic counselling (and we have seen that this happens all too rarely), the woman who awakens and finds that her breast has been removed is bound to be in a state of shock. This is true for every woman who has a mastectomy, whether or not she has been well prepared for it, and whether or not her breasts are especially important to her. A mastectomy is an amputation. While it doesn't deprive you of certain functional abilities as happens with the loss of a limb, its physical effect must not be under-estimated. Your body has been subjected to severe trauma and you need a little time, and much understanding to adjust to these physical effects as much as you need them to help you adjust mentally.

Every woman who has had a mastectomy knows the truth of these words and those who have not can make an effort to pro-ject themselves into the situation and correspondingly appreciate them. I express this fact so emphatically as much for the medical profession as for anyone, because although, in surgical terms, a mastectomy is usually a comparatively simple and straightforward operation, its combined physical and mental effects are no less traumatic for that. The women who are given sympathetic attention from their doctor, after the operation, and careful thoughtful nursing – even though they are not in a dramatic life-and-death situation – are going to recover faster and adjust better in every way to their new circumstances.

The intention of this book has been to promote positive, hopeful and helpful attitudes about the treatment of breast cancer. When so much good work is now being done it would be needlessly destructive to dwell on the unfortunate examples where this kind of attitude has been conspicuously lacking, more often due to sheer lack of imagination rather than deliberate unkindness or hardened indifference. Whatever the reasons, hospital staff should be aware that thoughtless words or behaviour at this crucial moment in a woman's life, when she has to come to terms with so much more than the knowledge that she has had a malignant tumour removed, can prove to have devastating, possibly irreversible effects on her long-term recovery. The remainder of this chapter is devoted to describing the best in post-operative care and physical aids that is now available and should be offered, as a matter of course, to every woman who has a mastectomy.

In hospital

Soon after the operation, you will be encouraged to start getting up and moving around, walking to the toilet and sitting in a chair. Apart from the minor awkwardness of having to carry drainage tubes around, which are fixed inside your stitches to take off any excess fluid, thus hastening the healing process, you may find that the arm of the operation side is uncomfortable if you let it hang down. You may also feel thrown off balance. 'Breasts are heavier than you think,' one medium-sized woman pointed out to me and said that it had surprised her how long it took to adjust to this shift in weight. If you have a big bosom this can be a real problem but it is very important to get it right quickly, otherwise your posture changes, resulting in muscular aches and pains elsewhere, a complication you can well do without.

Here are a couple of simple suggestions to cope with these difficulties which I have picked out of the American Reach to Recovery programme. This organization is now part of the American Cancer Society and all their exercises and recommendations are medically approved, but if your hospital doesn't know about them, it is wiser and certainly more tactful to ask your doctor's permission first.

1 An arm support

Ask the nurse or a visitor to roll up a towel or a strip of foam rubber into a sausage about 18 inches long and 6 inches thick which she then ties with a 2-inch bandage in three places. The two lengths of bandage should each be long enough to go diagonally across your chest and back and tie round your neck on your unaffected side. The roll is thus held against your body under your armpit and you can rest your aching arm on it. You will probably find it useful at home as well for the first few weeks until your arm has fully recovered.

2 Breast sling

To make this you need a piece of soft easily draped material about one and a quarter yards square, some large safety pins and a small firm pad of folded material roughly 4 inches square.

The nurse must help you by folding the material into a triangle and then, placing your breast comfortably into the middle of the triangle, she takes a slightly longer end under your breast and arm, round up your back and over your shoulder to meet the shorter end just above your breast. Instead of tying the sling which causes pressure because of the weight of your breast, she folds the two ends neatly and pins them together on top of the small pad. To give the sling a cup shape which will hold your breast firmly, she pins two more safety pins in the appropriate places to make the darts.

Again you may find this sling even more useful to wear at home when you are getting used to going about your daily chores and until you have had your permanent prosthesis fitted which should restore your balance.

Where the operation has been either a simple or a modified radical your scar will run neatly across your chest in a transverse line well below any low-necked dress or swim suit that you will want to wear later on. Providing that it heals well, you will be ready to go home between six and ten days after your operation. Until the time comes to take out your stitches your wound will be dressed regularly. Although this may sound very hard, it will help you in the long run if you can try to accustom yourself to looking downwards when the nurse does this so as to get used to the flatness. If you find this impossible, don't worry. Now is not the time to force yourself over too many hurdles and many women find this a particularly punishing one. Betty Westgate would like there to be a long mirror in every hospital bathroom so that those women who feel ready for it can make this first inspection quite on their own and before they go home where they may have other problems to face in this respect with their husband and possibly their children. Women who have a skin graft, due to more extensive surgery or because there is a problem with healing, will have to stay in hospital a little longer, while the new skin, usually taken from the thigh, settles down.

As soon as you begin to feel better in yourself, you should be doing some gentle exercising, under instruction from the physiotherapist, to mobilize your arm on the affected side. This is going to be painful to start with and you may wonder what the use of it is, but the sooner you can start exercising your stiff muscles, the less likelihood there is that they will shrink from lack of use, making it much more difficult for you to use your arm properly later on. These exercises must be done under careful medical supervision from your doctor but if nothing has been prescribed for you after the first few days, make a point of asking why. Some doctors are much more punctilious than others about this aspect of treatment but the old idea that the arm should be kept quite immobile for a fortnight has been totally superseded, unless of course your particular operation requires it. As long as you have stitches, you must obviously not be too energetic, but the physiotherapist should know exactly what you can and cannot do.

Looking good

In the last chapter I described how the clinical nurse consultant considered that fitting patients with their prosthesis was one of the most important aspects of her post-operative care.

She has done a lot of research into suitable bras, different types of prostheses and the shops which offer a special fitting service for mastectomies. Before the patient leaves the hospital she gives her a list of models and stockists. She also fits the patient with a lightweight foam rubber prosthesis which she can wear until her chest and scar have become less sensitive. In most cases, the woman can go home wearing the same bra as she wore before her operation and look the same. Exceptions are plunging and underwired ones, the former because they don't give enough support and the latter because they will press against her scar. When the patient comes back to the mastectomy clinic a few weeks later the nurse will then be able to advise her about her permanent prosthesis and under the National Health Service offer her a wide variety costing up to approximately £40. The patient does not pay for her prosthesis now or at any later date when she has to renew it. If, however, she finds nothing quite right for her, there are an increasing number on the market and the nurse will be able to tell her where to go, even give her the name of a specially trained fitter.

Unfortunately, few hospitals have this kind of person in charge of appliance fitting, as it is called, and all too often the appliance officer is a man. Now he may be perfectly nice and as concerned to do his best for mastectomy patients as for anyone else he meets on his round, but it seems to me quite unlikely that he can ever be as sympathetic and sensitive, in what is a very delicate situation, in the way that another woman could be. How can he be? He has never had breasts. He doesn't know anything about buying bras in normal circumstances and the women with whom he comes into contact in their hospital beds are struggling to cope with circumstances which are far from normal. It's hardly a time to be greeted with the cheery cry of 'Let me be your bosom friend' as one was quoted in a *Guardian* article recently.

Many hospitals are extremely offhand about the whole business, still offering a very limited range of prostheses and no real advice about how to wear them. Some are even unaware that the days of birdseed bags and inert shapeless lumps which have an unnerving habit of dropping out of the bra when the woman bends over are long since gone. Such attitudes spring, I suspect, from the example given by the type of surgeon who can say, as one did to a woman who has worked for years travelling round the country as a mastectomy fitter: 'Hmm. I suppose you're one of these females who go around telling ladies to ask for these,' while disdainfully picking up one of the latest models in breast forms, to which, I am glad to say, she retorted with a spirited, 'Yes, you bet I am.' Is it any wonder, therefore, that Dr Maguire's research has revealed that one-third of mastectomy patients are deeply dissatisfied with the prostheses that they have been given? This is an inexcusable situation, given that good ones are now available on the National Health.

June Marchant, who had a mastectomy herself, was so disturbed by the depth of ignorance and indifference on this subject which exists in so many hospitals that she has gone to enormous pains to research everything that is available, both in bras and prostheses, to suit every type of mastectomy patient. Her results, which list every important detail, including sizes, prices and stockists, and a wealth of other practical advice which doctors and nurses as well as women could read with profit, have been published in an excellent paperback (see bibliography). Rather than attempt to repeat her effort, which I could only offer in an abbreviated form, I suggest that this little book is a worthwhile buy for any woman who is at a loss to know where or how to start looking.

Self-help

Another invaluable source of information and guidance comes from the Mastectomy Association (address in the Appendix).

This is another self-help effort from another mastectomee, Betty Westgate, who founded her organization six years ago when she realized just how badly women were in need of help, particularly when they left the cocooned atmosphere of the hospital ward and found themselves trying to resume a normal life. Her leaflet, 'Helpful Hints' is distributed free to mastectomy patients in every hospital which will accept them. She is personally responsible for inspiring bra manufacturers to produce new lines especially for the mastectomee and urging medical appliance companies to develop new and more convincing types of prosthesis. Among the best is one made of a silicone gel which moulds itself to the chest wall. It has a natural shape and a soft movement under the most clinging dress or skinniest jumper, and for a little extra you can buy one with a nipple. Mrs Westgate will send free comprehensive details about all these products, including makes of swimwear and nightdresses, to anyone who writes to her, but you should enclose a stamp.

Possibly the most valuable service she offers lies with her army of volunteers, now some 1,500 strong, who are all mastectomees and who live in every part of Britain. These women are available at the end of a telephone line or they will make a home visit to any woman who has just had a mastectomy and wants help and advice. She doesn't know them all personally but they come to her with a recommendation, many through doctors who do approve of the work being done by her association. She matches the volunteer carefully in age and social circumstances to the woman who is seeking aid but she stresses that the advice they give is strictly non-medical and they are not encouraged to be amateur psychologists. Fundamentally, what they are offering is practical information and the reassurance that only someone who has lived through the same experience can give. She says that one talk is usually enough and the fact that the women are strangers to each other and remain that way is very important. The volunteers don't encourage self-pity and indeed most women don't want to harp on their misfortunes, but if a caller does seem very upset and in need of more skilled help than the volunteer is qualified to give, she rings in to Mrs Westgate who will then put the woman in touch with the appropriate professional person in her area. She has made an agreement with the medical profession that she will never organize group meetings but doubts whether they would be very successful anyway. In her view the healthy attitude to breast cancer is to put it firmly in the past. You can't forget that you have had it, but you can stop thinking about it, if other people will let you. This sentiment was repeated to me many times by other women. As one said, 'talking of survival doesn't please me one inch. It's how you live the time you have to live which matters', a truth which surely every one of us could take to heart.

At home

Betty Westgate, and possibly there are others like her, is making a valiant attempt to plug the gaps left by the professionals, but why do they exist and why are there so many? For instance, few women are told about the simple exercises which they can do at home to improve mobility of their arm. Nor are they always told about certain precautions that they must take to avoid infection and swelling, particularly if they have had a radical operation which means that their lymph glands have been removed and consequently their immune resistance has been lowered. Radiotherapy can also cause this uncomfortable condition.

A simple leaflet issued to every woman before she leaves hospital wouldn't take too much of anyone's time and could prevent a host of troublesome difficulties and possible complications later on. Lymphoedema, unfortunately, cannot always be averted, but it can be alleviated. Here are a few tips from the Reach to Recovery programme which could usefully be incorporated in any such advice.

Arm exercises

These should be done in the following order and on the principle of a little at a time. Never strain yourself but make a point of reaching a little further and a little longer each time you do them. Remember that it is always the arm on your operation side which is being exercised. Ask for your doctor's advice before you start them.

1 *Hair brushing*
Prop your arm on a pile of books placed on your dressing table. Sit straight, hold your head up and start brushing one side of your head. Gradually work all the way round, possibly at different times until you are able to brush all your hair.

2 *Newspaper crumpling*
Place a pile of separated newspaper pages on a table and rest your arm from elbow to wrist on it. Crumple the pages completely, one by one. Squeezing a soft rubber ball in your hand, which you can do at any time of the day (in a standing position), has the same effect of strengthening the hand and arm muscles.

3 *Walking up the wall*
Stand with feet apart (flat shoes or barefoot), facing the wall with your forehead resting against it. Gradually reach upwards with your hands pressing lightly against it. Do this slowly and often, but don't overtax yourself. Eventually you will be able to reach right above your head with your arms straight.

4 *Rope swinging*
Tie a length of rope round a door handle. Stand or sit at right angles to it, holding the other end in your affected hand lightly but firmly. Start swinging it gently in small circles, gradually making them bigger as your arm becomes more flexible.

As you get more practised you can devise other exercises for yourself, based on the same reaching principle but do remember not to over-do it. There are also several household chores which use the same muscles, like hanging up the washing, reaching up to a top shelf or cleaning the windows. What you must avoid is lifting anything heavy or pushing or pulling. Typing and knitting are also good exercises.

Precautions
1 If you have had radiotherapy or develop lymphoedema – *never* allow your arm to be vaccinated, injected, sampled for blood or tested for blood pressure.

2 Protect your hand and arm against cuts, burns and scrapes. Wear loose-fitting gloves whenever possible for household chores – oven gloves for handling hot dishes, kitchen gloves for washing clothes and dishes, and heavy-duty ones for work in the garden.

3 Protect your arm against sunburn.

4 Don't cut your cuticles.

5 Wear a thimble for sewing.

If you develop an infection, however slight, see your doctor immediately as prompt action could spare you considerable and sometimes lasting discomfort.

To avoid lymphoedema keep your arm supported as much as possible. At night you can sleep with it on a pillow, holding it above your head. At least you can start off with it in that position. Should lymphoedema develop you must see your doctor, who may decide to treat it with antibiotics. There are also ways you can help yourself, but get your doctor's agreement first. Crêpe bandaging at night or wearing an elastic sleeve are two methods. The aim is to support but not to constrict. It is also possible to reduce the swelling by using a mechanical pump and sleeve but you should only do this on medical advice.

Expect the first few weeks after the operation to be frustrating and difficult at times. You will tire easily and temporary handicaps brought about by your stiff muscles can assume undue proportions. However, if you have a job, it is a good idea to go back to it as soon as you feel strong enough because the stimulus provided by your work and workmates will help you to forget your own problems. The mother with young children will also be distracted by the constant attention she must give to them but it may be harder for the woman who is usually alone at home during the day. Whoever you are, you probably won't want to fling yourself immediately into a mad social whirl, but equally don't shrink away from your friends or usual activities.

Ease yourself back into your old life. It hasn't come to a full stop because of your illness, but there has been a pause and it has changed.

14 Your life

Life will never be the same again, cries the woman who has had breast cancer and it's true for her, as it's true for everyone in different ways at different times. Life changes all the time. Life changes us and our life changes the lives of others. We can't escape our human condition and the more deeply we are committed to living and loving in all its aspects – people, work, politics, pleasure – all that absorbs and fulfils us, the more vulnerable we are to loss. Sickness, accidents and death threaten us all. They are the price we pay for living and sooner or later the toll is exacted from each and every one of us. Breast cancer is an especially cruel demand on any woman of any age in any circumstances. As one who has not had to meet it I have no right to suggest to women who have, how they should respond to it. Everything that follows, therefore, is based on the experiences of women who, having journeyed through this dark valley, are willing to write or talk about it because they care for other women who may one day have to face the same ordeal.

A woman tends to think of herself first in relation to others, and only secondly, if at all, as a person in her own right. Now that may be all wrong, and the women's movement suggests strongly that it is, and possibly the women who follow us will reverse that attitude, or at least balance it better, but the fact remains that that is how most women today see themselves. And it is in that light that they have to face their personal future after a mastectomy.

The married woman thinks immediately of her husband's reaction. How will he take it? How can she return to him, a damaged article, no longer the woman he fell in love with and married? Won't he find her repulsive and unlovable? How can he bear to make love to 'half a woman'?

These fears are often unspoken but rather than face his

rejection she rejects him before he has had a chance to deny them and prove that his love hasn't changed. It would be foolish to pretend that even the most mature and firm relationship between a husband and wife is not going to be rocked by this event, but they have had other crises in their life which they have surmounted together and there is no reason, providing they talk this one out, that they cannot do the same again and probably come through it, stronger and more loving and grateful for each other than before.

'As long as she's here, it doesn't worry me what bits and pieces are missing,' one man said to me, and turning to his wife, added, 'You know that. I've told you time and time again.' Theirs was an unaffectedly happy marriage which had survived exceptionally difficult times with illness, tragic accidents and other family disasters attacking them on all sides, but it seemed that each new blow had the effect of cementing rather than threatening their relationship.

A woman in a good marriage is a lucky woman but other wives and other husbands will need more help from each other, and possibly from outsiders too, if they are to survive the tremors caused by her illness. Some men do mind about the mutilation and are not able to accept it. Some women are so haunted by what has happened to them that they just cannot recover their former spirit and fight the depression and unhappiness which invades them. They need continuing support if they are to pull through together and sometimes they don't. A few marriages do founder but if it had not been this crisis, probably another would have caused the same damage. Sometimes a break-up can even be for the best as this woman felt about hers. 'Two terrible things happened to me in the same year. My husband died and I got breast cancer but today I can truthfully say that I am a better and a happier woman.' She has found a man who loves her for the whole woman she is, and a marvellous job, and she feels that her future has never been so exciting.

The single woman, whether she be divorced, widowed or unmarried, tends to be unfairly left out when it comes to getting the sympathy hand-outs. One woman in her thirties reported to me that when her doctor discovered that she was not married, he remarked casually, 'well, you're all right, then'. His assumption that she had no man in her life to worry about, either then or was likely to have in the future, both enraged and terrified her. Perhaps he was right, she thought, she was going to turn into a titless freak, a monster from whom all men would recoil. Another woman who expressed similar fears to a woman friend recounts with bitter-sweet amusement the response which was supposed to reassure her: 'Oh, don't worry about that! I know someone like you who's found a lover with only one leg.' In other words, freaks unite!

Fortunately, not everybody meets quite such thoughtless reactions, but there is one aching problem which remains for every single woman who does want to have a sexual relationship. When should she tell? Some women get it out at once before there is the faintest suggestion of interest in the man's eyes, giving him the chance to retreat fast before there can be any hurt feelings. Others find it has a permanently inhibiting effect on their relationships because they get so far and then, their nerve failing them, they hastily put on the dampers, leaving a trail of frustrated angry men who wonder why they've been turned down. It's rather like the old days when a woman had to decide when and whether to confess that she had lost her virginity. One woman, who says that she has had the two best love affairs of her life after her mastectomy, feels that 'it is a risk you just have to take each time. If he's going to run out on you, better now than later on.' If you love a man, it seems only fair to give him at least the chance to prove how much he can love you in return.

Undressing in front of their husband or lover is probably the major hurdle women face. It may take them months before they can allow themselves to be seen in the bath or walking around the bedroom. The man may need to take the initiative here. He must use every ploy he can think of to convince her that he wants her, and that with or without a breast she is the same woman for him. Many men find it difficult to put into words what they genuinely think and feel, but this is a time when they must overcome their diffidence. If necessary, they should seek help from a professional source, like a marriage guidance counsellor who can give practical advice based on the individual circumstances.

Children also have to be considered. When and how to tell them and whether to show yourself naked to them depends in part on your family habits, in part on their age and their individual characters. 'Never force anything on them until they are ready for it,' advises one mother who used a different approach towards each of her three children. The curiosity of the inquisitive child should be satisfied. The silence of another should be respected but at the same time gently encouraged to be broken. One thing you can be certain of from your children is that they are not going to stop loving you. You are the same mother, just much more precious.

Who to tell? is another problem which worries some women enormously and others not at all. The taboos on talking about breast cancer have broken down very much in the last few years since many women in the public eye have announced their operation to a fanfare of publicity and with the expressed hope that their frankness will inspire other women to look after themselves better and to seek help, if they need it, earlier. Actually, the Americans do this much more readily than we taciturn British but the more women who can say openly, yes, I have had it and here I am ten, fifteen or whatever years later, perfectly all right, the better chance there is that more women will take their cancers early for treatment. Again, however, this is very much a matter of personal preference and no woman should feel obliged to announce to all and sundry that she has just lost a breast. Sometimes it is easier to tell strangers than it is to tell your own close family, particularly someone like your mother, whose concern for you may be more than you can bear. It is very important in this matter of telling that the woman herself should do it. It is her body and it is her decision who she wants to know about it. Well-meaning friends and relatives who go around with long faces, blurting out the bad news in a stage whisper do more harm than they realize. No woman wants to see ill-disguised concern and that stare of macabre curiosity so many people seem unable to refrain from when they hear 'it's cancer'.

'I'm going to go on living until I die,' exulted one friend of mine. To have been touched by death, she says, was the best lesson of her life. Now that she has sorted out her priorities and wiped out superficial relationships – 'I've got no time to waste' – she intends to enjoy every minute that she has.

An intimation of mortality brushes every woman who has had breast cancer but can any of us escape such feelings at some time in our life? The death of a parent, a spouse or a dearly loved friend fills us with a sense of loss and regret while it reminds us of the frailty of our own lives. The death of a child is a ravaging grief for its parents which they find harder to bear than any illness they may have. Breast cancer is a cruel disease, but there are others which bring more pain and more disfigurement and greater loss of function. The suffering caused by mental illness can seem more impossible to overcome than almost any physical affliction. People every day are struck by worse adversity. Many women say that this particular crisis brings happiness with it as well as sadness. They are moved by the deeper warmth and fresh tenderness it arouses in their intimate relationships and the kindness that it sparks from people who have formerly been on the edge of their lives.

The woman who has had breast cancer hopes that she will live as long as any woman of her age is entitled to expect. There is always a chance that the disease may recur, but if it does, it can be controlled. It has not yet been conquered but, as we have seen, there is a well-founded hope for the future that more and more women will be permanently cured. That is not a pious wish but a definite promise. Meanwhile, let us be sustained by the examples of courage and blithe defiance shown to us by so many women who have had it. They are whole women, real women, who have been enriched and extended by their experience.

Postscript

In my introduction to the first edition of this book I expressed the hope that it would be completely out of date in ten years time. I was thinking in particular of the various orthodox medical treatments that women diagnosed with breast cancer can now expect to receive: surgery, radiotherapy, chemotherapy and endocrine therapy, to name the most important; sometimes one on its own, but more often administered conjointly or serially, over a period of years. I didn't think then, and I don't think now, that some or all of these treatments can ever be entirely superseded, at least not until the day arrives when we fully understand the causes of cancer, which will enable us to take the appropriate preventive measures well in advance of the disease appearing.

However, when it came to reviewing the situation three years later, I was ready to face the author's nightmare of having to re-write parts of the book if it meant being able to mention any major developments which could spell new hope for women but, as I scanned the medical literature and made my enquiries among those working in the field, it began to look as if I would be hard pressed to find anything at all of note to add. True, there are many more trials under way, but statistics have yet to be measured and conclusions to be drawn. Certain treatments such as adjuvant chemotherapy at the time of treating the primary breast cancer with the aim of destroying any micro-metastases which may have lodged themselves in other parts of the body look even more promising now than they did then. There is some encouraging new data about the value of early screening. More doctors in the National Health Service are offering implants. The search for a reliable biochemical test to aid early screening and for a 'tumour marker' to determine the extent of a returning malignancy and consequently, the type and degree of further treatment, continues.

All in all, progress on the medical front is characterised by inches, not strides. There are no dramatic break-throughs to report, and no marvellous wonder-drug has emerged. It is debatable whether we should even expect one but as yet there is not even a glimmer of evidence on which to base a hope that doctors and scientists may be close to a solution. Meanwhile, this vicious enemy of women is, if anything, becoming more rampant and aggressive. The annual toll continues to rise inexorably, particularly in the developed Western world, and I personally continue to hear chilling stories of the indifference to their psychological needs and the overwhelming sense of isolation that so many women have to suffer in the course of their treatment. Regretfully, I have to admit that the factual content of this book remains as relevant and as up-to-date in all but details as it was when first I wrote it.

And yet, despite these gloomy facts, I believe that today we have more reason to feel optimistic about the future than ever before. Materially, the situation may not have changed all that much, but spiritually, and I introduce this term deliberately into a clinical context, I believe there have been significant advances. Many more doctors are asking themselves and discussing with their colleagues whether automatic mastectomy on a diagnosis of breast cancer is always necessary. The long-term survival rates show that there is no difference in the ultimate outcome of the disease whatever the form of early treatment, whether it be radical or simple mastectomy, lumpectomy with or without radiotherapy, or radiotherapy on its own. Breast cancer is a systemic disease which means that by the time a lump is discovered in the breast it is highly likely that cancer cells will have been shed, via the bloodstream, in other parts of the body. If the lymph nodes are involved, then it is 100 per cent certain, and additional systemic therapy is essential.

The two main arguments in favour of mastectomy for an early breast cancer are, firstly, that by removing the entire breast the surgeon can be certain that he has removed other potential or actual cancer sites in the breast itself, and, secondly, that by so doing, he has almost entirely eliminated the risk of local recurrence. A third important argument, which is valid only in those treatment centres where it is now recognised that further adjuvant therapy may be required at an early stage to destroy as yet undiscovered micro-metastases, is that the larger the sample of tumour and surrounding tissue the better chance there is to determine the biological properties of the tumour, and, consequently, the type of treatment required. For one woman it could be cytotoxic drugs; for another, it could be hormonal; and there are other possibilities. The reasoning behind these arguments is described at greater length in chapters 8 and 10.

My purpose in raising the issue here is to emphasise, perhaps more strongly than I did originally, that there is absolutely no place any longer for what one cancer specialist has called 'mindless mastectomies', in other words surgery performed as an automatic response to presentation of a malignant breast lump. The patient's total condition must be very carefully examined and considered – and discussed with her – before deciding on treatment, and this can really only happen in hospitals where there is a medical team which, in addition to pooling its members' skills and exchanging information about their own work, is also keeping abreast of developments in other centres, here and abroad.

This move towards a more open-minded consideration of all the available treatment options is supported by a growing realisation, certainly among younger doctors, that to be jealous of preserving one's own particular expertise, come what may in the shape of new knowledge, and at the expense of underestimating or even excluding alternatives from other disciplines, is, to say the least, to fall short of professional excellence. Even more important, for humanitarian reasons, is the danger that such a narrow-minded approach may well deprive patients of their right to receive the best, most appropriate medical care for their specific condition. The signs are that these progressive attitudes are slowly gaining ground and turning into accepted practice but, unhappily, they are still not nearly as widespread as they should be. Worsening economic stringencies in the National Health Service do not encourage a radical re-organisation of resources, and we still have to wait for a whole generation of diehard doctors, stuck in the mould of outdated techniques and thinking they learnt in medical school thirty or forty years ago and have never since paused to question, to disappear before we can be sure that every woman with breast cancer will get the carefully considered, individual treatment she needs.

So what, if any, advances are there to report?

It is always easier to explain fundamental shifts in thinking after they have happened. The process of gradual enlightenment which slowly guides towards altered attitudes and finally translates into new action is subtle and elusive of documentation. There is, however, one important trend now surfacing which only a short time ago was being dismissed at best as opinion unsupported by facts and at worst as dangerously wishful thinking. The arguments for a conservative approach to breast cancer surgery have for some time had their few brave advocates in the medical profession, who, for their pains, have been subjected to a barrage of hostile contempt, or quite simply ignored.

At this point I would like to make good an omission in the book and acknowledge the pioneering work of Sir Geoffrey Keynes, who, as a surgeon at St Bartholomew's Hospital in London fifty years ago, was probably the first doctor to reject radical mastectomy, denouncing it as a 'futile mutilation'. Instead he used either limited surgery or a form of radium therapy which consisted of inserting radium needles into the tumour. Today, both interstitial radioactive implants (irridium wires threaded through the tumour requiring hospitalisation for only a few days) and external irradiation therapy is being offered as an alternative to mastectomy for women with *early* breast cancer at many centres in Europe and North America. In the book I reflect the doubts expressed in the medical papers extant at the time about the ultimate external appearance of the breast. Today, there is new evidence in a paper by Drs Martinez and

Goffinet at Stanford, California, that enhanced techniques now make it possible to achieve excellent and lasting cosmetic results. Furthermore, the well-worn criticism that this alternative to mastectomy is unsupported by adequate follow-up studies is no longer valid. There is now plenty of hard evidence to support the view expressed by Dr Fletcher and others in 1976 'that women with early breast cancer take no chance on their life by having a treatment method which preserves the breast'.

British medical opinion remains cautious about the possibility of supplanting mastectomy altogether in favour of radiotherapy. But at least more doctors are thinking about it and several trials comparing the two forms of treatment are now under way. Lumpectomy combined with radiotherapy is also being offered more readily to those patients for whom it seems appropriate, which is by no means always the case.

Another hopeful development related to breast conservation is that women who ask for an implant after mastectomy are no longer automatically treated as vain silly creatures with no right to be demanding psychological supports of this kind. Three years ago it was almost impossible to get an implant after mastectomy on the National Health Service. Today, there are many hospitals where a woman can discuss, without fear of derision, her suitability for this operation. Many doctors will advise her to wait a few months, even a year or two before having it done and the reasons for this advice may not be entirely medical, although it must be said in this respect that there can be problems of matching the new breast with the old. The evidence from a recent study conducted in Edinburgh by Professor Forrest and Dr Christine Dean (a psychiatrist) shows that the main benefit from an immediate reconstruction is that it gives women more self-confidence and freedom to wear what they like. For some women, particularly those who had admitted beforehand to having a rocky marriage, the psychological benefits were also striking.

I have already mentioned that early adjuvant chemotherapy seems to reduce the recurrence rate for some women. The joint American/Italian trial to which I refer in chapter 10 has now been completed and shows that for post-menopausal node-positive women on a drug-regimen combining L-phenylaline mustard and 5-fluorouracil (PF) the recurrence rate after two years has been reduced from 45 per cent to 30 per cent. When this treatment was supplemented by tamoxifen (an anti-oestrogen) it went down to 5 per cent, a fact which emphasises how vital it is to establish at the time of biopsy whether the tumour is hormone-dependent. The advantage of tamoxifen is that it has virtually no side effects and trials are now going on in this country to see whether it can be used for node-negative as well as node-positive women.

Until recently endocrine or hormone therapy involving the removal of the ovaries has been regarded as effective for delaying recurrence for some pre-menopausal women and also for slowing down the advance of secondaries, but not for bettering ultimate survival. Now, however, Dr Meakin's study from Toronto (reported in 1980) indicates that it may make a significant difference to survival as well when combined with a drug called prednisone.

There is one point on which everyone is in agreement: the earlier the cancer is detected, the better the woman's chance of making a complete recovery. But the debate still revolves on such issues as how best to apply mammography (now accepted as the most reliable diagnostic technique) how often, to what women and the extent of risk they run from ionising radiation. The thorny question of cost-effectiveness is also unresolved.

Professor Baum, in his book *Breast Cancer, The Facts (OUP 1981)* estimates on the basis of some complicated and, as he himself admits, 'unverifiable assumptions' that the cost of saving one woman's life picked up in a screening programme could be as high as £40,000. He also remarks on the significant number of women who will refuse an invitation to screening because they are fearful of the outcome. His views are not supported by the information which has come out of a two-year screening study in Sweden which was carried out on a combined urban and rural population of 37,640 women. The average participation rate was 82 per cent (the oldest women were least inclined to

attend) and it climbed to 92 per cent for those women aged
between 40 (the lower age limit) and 70 who constituted the
major proportion of women invited. The costs of running the
programme, which was carried out with a mobile unit, were very
low: £4.40 for every woman invited, rising to £5.40 for those
who accepted examination. (This is cheaper than a cervical
smear programme which was being carried out at the same
time.) Of the 367 women who were referred from screening for
further investigation, 127 were finally proved to have cancer and
the cost of treating these patients varied between £1320 and
£1500, depending on the nature of the cancer. It is true that
these figures do not take into account further expenses if the
patient suffers a recurrence nor do they include the overall costs
of future bi- or tri-annual screening which is necessary for a
totally efficient screening programme, but they fall far short of
the dizzy sums suggested by Professor Baum.

These Swedish results will have important implications for the
Department of Health and Social Security when it takes stock of
its own screening trials, now nearly halfway through their eight-
year term, (see chapter 5). Preliminary results from their
screening centres suggest that breast cancers are being diagnosed at an early stage and that women are responding well to
the invitation to participate.

So much for what the doctors and the cancer researchers are
doing – more perhaps than we realise – but is there also more
that women can do to help themselves and each other? The
Women's National Cancer Control Campaign, which has done
so much to promote cervical examinations and education in
breast self-examination, now needs informed, determined
backing from women's organisations in its demand for an
intelligent and sympathetic evaluation of the accumulating evidence in favour of screening for breast cancer.

Screening is not the same as prevention and until we know
what causes breast cancer it is difficult to recommend specific
preventive measures. Monthly breast self-examination is,
however, essential; a habit that every woman should assume as
part of her self-care routine. Attention to diet is sensible. There

is a definite correlation between a high fat diet and certain cancers, in particular cancer of the colon and of the breast. This may be because animal fats deposited in the system produce a more favourable environment for developing latent tumour cells. A new line of research suggests that there may also be a link between chronic constipation and breast cancer, possibly due to bacteria acting on food in the constipated bowel to transform ordinary cells into cancer cells. It is known that bacteria in the bowel produce female hormones, especially among women eating a lot of meat and fat. Constipation may cause these superfluous hormones to be reabsorbed and stimulate the growth of breast cancer cells. It improves looks as well as health in general to adopt what the Americans call the Prudent Diet by cutting down on fatty meats, dairy products, sugar, and refined flour and grain products, substituting them with plenty of fresh vegetables, fruit and whole grain foods which are rich in proteins, minerals, vitamins and the fibre to stimulate daily bowel action.

The mind is part of the body and plays a vital role in regeneration and resistance. This may seem obvious to those who have always maintained that there is a place for alternative therapies in the treatment of disease, but many more orthodox doctors are now coming round to this view. A new study of breast cancer patients, done by the psychological unit at King's College Hospital, London, shows that those women who were determined to fight their disease survived longer and did better than their more passive and resigned sisters. The 'good' patient, that is to say the one who accepts without question what is offered to her, may not always be doing what is best for her. The Cancer Research Campaign is sufficiently impressed by these results to be funding a new trial to compare two groups of cancer patients: those receiving orthodox treatment alone, with those who will get additional psychological support in the form of group therapy or meditation. This view is endorsed by the recently formed *Association for New Approaches to Cancer* (1a Addison Crescent, London W14 8JP. Tel. 01-603 7751) which includes doctors as well as alternative therapists among its members. It emphasises that its aim is not to oust orthodox treatments, but to make people aware that there are alternatives which may, without raising false hopes, improve their mental state and certainly will not inflict the drastic physical side-effects of so much orthodox treatment.

When I was first researching for this book a prominent doctor in the field suddenly expostulated to me: 'I can't understand why you women haven't been making more fuss about the treatment you get for breast cancer. If you had, we might have started sooner to wonder why the methods we have practised almost unchanged for decades have been so dreadfully unsuccessful in controlling this disease.' He is something of an exception in his profession, even today. Now that women are raising their voices, are coming out of the cancer closet of shame and fear, are questioning what is meted out to them and requesting information about alternatives, there are many doctors who wish they would just shut up and go away. There are dark mutterings about therapeutic anarchy and feminist incitement to medical mayhem. Sounds lurid? Maybe, but that is what is being said in some quarters by doctors who are angered by what they see as a threat to their professional standing. Yet I doubt whether there would now be so many trials going on to compare, for example, conservative alternatives to mastectomy, were it not for all those brave women who have spoken up about their own experiences, some of whom have proceeded to positive action to help other women: Rose Kushner, for instance, in America, who has set up a Cancer Enquiry Service, and Betty Westgate and others in this country who are organising mastectomy support groups.

What we need now is a genuine spirit of co-operation between the health professionals, the alternative health therapists and all those who seek their help. Informed women informing other women is the best way we can help each other. If this book has helped you in any way to gain a better understanding of breast cancer, please pass on your knowledge to a friend who may not want to read it for herself, but needs the information.

Carolyn Faulder, London 1982

Glossary

Adenoma – a benign tumour.

Adjuvant – auxiliary or additional. Term applied to any therapy which is used as back-up to primary treatment (usually surgery) of primary tumour. Chemotherapy, radiotherapy and hormone therapy can all be used as adjuvants.

Adrenal Glands – two small organs near the kidneys which are responsible for synthesizing and releasing several hormones, primarily catecholamines and steroids.

Aetiology – science of the causes of disease.

Axilla – armpit, hence **Axillary** – relating to the armpit.

Benign – medical term for describing condition which is mild and non-malignant but may require treatment.

Biopsy – the surgical removal of a small piece of tissue for laboratory examination by a pathologist to determine whether it is malignant. **Excision Biopsy** is surgical removal of the whole lump.

Carcinogen – any agent which causes cancer.

Carcinoma – a malignant tumour arising in tissue which forms the outer layer of body surface or lining of cavities that open to the body surface. This tissue (called epithelial) includes skin, glands, nerves, breasts and the linings of the respiratory, gastro-intestinal, urinary and genital systems. Carcinomas account for approximately 85 per cent of human cancers.

Carcinoma in Situ – often also called **Pre-Invasive Carcinoma**. This means that the tumour is contained within its place of origin and has not spread. Removing it at this localized stage offers a very high chance of cure.

Chemotherapy – the use of one or more anti-cancer (cytotoxic) drugs to destroy cancer cells which have spread from the primary tumour to other parts of the body. If used when cancer is first diagnosed, known as **Adjuvant Chemotherapy** (see **Adjuvant** above).
Combination Chemotherapy describes the use of several anti-cancer

drugs in varying proportions to treat early and advanced cancer. This is based on the principle that their combined use will improve their effectiveness and reduce toxicity.

Clinical medicine is medical practice based on observed symptoms. Hence **Clinical Examination** for breast disease is the physical examination of a patient's breast and **Clinical Staging** is diagnosing the extent of cancer by analysing the conclusions drawn from the examination.

Cyst – an accumulation of material, usually fluid, contained in a sac. It is a common non-malignant swelling and it is only very rarely associated with a cancer.

Cytotoxic – anti-cancer. Term applied to the drugs used in chemotherapy.

Endocrine or Hormone therapy – treatment controlling hormone activity in tumours suspected to be hormone-dependent.

Endogenous – growing or originating from within the body.

Epidemiology – science of epidemics and now of disease generally.

Exogenous – growing or originating from outside the body.

Frozen Section – small piece of suspect tissue which is cut out (excised) at biopsy, frozen and sent for immediate pathological examination.

Gamma Rays – a type of electromagnetic radiation with wavelengths shorter than those of X-rays. They, therefore, carry more energy than X-rays and when used for radiotherapy deliver more energy to tumours, except for those X-rays now delivered by a linear accelerator which has energies of several million volts.

Histology – science of organic tissues, hence **Histologic Analysis** is examining tissue for changes caused by disease and **Histologic Classification** is naming and determining the extent and type of disease.

Hormone – a chemical substance, produced in certain parts of the body, which has a specific effect on the activity of one or more distant organs.

Hormone Replacement Therapy (HRT) – usually refers to treatment of menopausal and post-menopausal women who are given oestrogen by tablet, injection or implant to replace the oestrogen deficiency which is the natural result of the ovaries ceasing to function.

Immunology – a scientific study of resistance to infection in humans and animals. Hence **Immunological** responses describe ways by which

the body defends itself against disease; **Immunosuppressive** refers to
any agent which prevents these defence mechanisms from operating;
and **Immunotherapy** is treatment based on principle of supporting
or improving the body's natural defence mechanisms.

Implant – artificial substance, usually silicone gel, which is inserted
into breast cavity to replace the natural breast.

Ionizing radiation – energy emitted as electromagnetic waves.
Is used in radiotherapy and X-ray diagnosis. Must be used
with care as heavy or too many repeated applications can
cause cancer.

Lesion – change in the functioning or texture of an organ which is
caused by disease.

Local Recurrence – cancer which reappears on site of original tumour.
Hence **Local Therapy** is treatment applied directly to this site.

Lumpectomy – the most conservative form of mastectomy
involving removal of malignant tumour only in the breast
together with surrounding tissue.

Lymph – colourless fluid from body tissue and organs which resembles
blood but has no red corpuscles.

Lymphangioma – a benign tumour arising in lymph vessels.

Lymph Gland or **Node** – small mass of tissue where lymph is purified
and lymphocytes are formed. In breast cancer, the condition of the
axillary, pectoral and mammary nodes which surround the breast is
an important indication for prognosis about the extent of cancer
spread.

Lymphocyte – a form of **Leucocyte** which is a colourless blood cell
also in lymph.

Lymphoedema – swelling of the arm caused by fluid which is unable
to drain away normally because the lymphatic drainage system, i.e. the
lymph nodes, have been surgically removed.

Malignant – in cancer refers to growths which will spread with
potentially fatal results if not removed.

Mamma or **Mammary Gland** – milk-secreting organ of female
mammals; in women called the breast.

Mammography – X-ray diagnostic technique specially
developed to investigate the breast for cancer cells.

Mastectomy – surgical procedure to remove the whole breast.

Menarche – first menstruation.

Menopause – period of life, usually between 45 to 55, when a woman ceases to menstruate, signifying the end of her reproductive life.

Metastasis – the process by which malignant cells detach themselves from the primary tumour and establish themselves in distant parts of the body, starting new tumours, called **Metastases or Secondaries.**

Morbidity – diseased state of organ or tissue.

Neoplasia – cancer.

Neoplasm – malignant tumour.

Neoplastic – of, or relating to, malignant tumours.

Node-positive – describes condition of one or more lymph nodes diagnosed as invaded by cancer cells.

Nulliparous – refers to woman who has never given birth.

Occult Carcinoma – a small tumour which is asymptomatic (gives no indication of its presence).

Oncology – the study of the causes, development, characteristics and treatment of cancer.

Oopherectomy – procedure, either by surgery or radiation, to remove the ovaries, sometimes called **Castration.**

Pituitary Gland, also known as the **Hypophysis** – a small organ situated at the base of the brain which is responsible for synthesizing and releasing at least nine different hormones. Exerts important influence on growth and bodily functions.

Prognosis – medical prediction about the development of a disease diagnosed in a patient.

Prolactin – hormone secreted by the pituitary gland which stimulates the milk flow.

Prophylactic – medical action to prevent disease.

Prosthesis – artificial part to replace some portion of the human anatomy. Where there has been a mastectomy, the term applies equally to surgical implants and to breast forms, made of various materials, which are put into the empty bra cup.

Radiotherapy – treatment of cancer by ionizing radiation which is energy emitted as electromagnetic waves to destroy the malignant cells. In early cancer the aim is to remove all malignancy; in advanced cancer this is no longer possible but it is palliative, i.e. it temporarily lessens the effects of the disease.

Radium – radioactive metallic element derived from pitchblende which is sometimes used in radiotherapy.

Remission – a period of good health occurring after the onset of cancer which can happen spontaneously or be induced by therapy.

Screening Programme – large-scale study of women invited to present themselves for breast examination to check for cancer. Various methods may be used, severally or singly.

Secondaries – recurrence of cancer cells in distant parts of the body after discovery of the primary tumour.

Steroids – large group of organic compounds including cholesterol, the sex hormones and the D-vitamins among others. Some steroids can be used as anti-cancer agents.

Systemic – refers to the body as a whole system. Hence **Systemic Therapy** is treatment aiming to attack malignancy wherever it may be throughout the body.

Tumour – swelling mass of tissue in any part of the body, derived from pre-existing cells, which serves no purpose and grows independently of surrounding tissue. **Benign tumours** remain localized, are usually slow growing and only produce symptoms when their size interferes with surrounding tissue. **Malignant tumours** have varying rates of growth but eventually, if left untreated, they tend to invade surrounding tissue and spread to other parts of the body.

Appendix

Full screening for breast cancer (including mammography and sometimes thermography as well) is not yet generally available on the National Health Service. However, many Local Authority Family Planning and Well Woman Clinics which screen for cervical cancer do a manual examination of the breasts at the same time and give instruction in breast self-examination. The Women's National Cancer Control Campaign (address on page 143) keeps an up-to-date list of all such clinics and will advise you which one is nearest to you.

Diagnostic facilities vary greatly from region to region, but if you want to know what is available and in which hospital in your area, contact your local Area Health Authority. The address and telephone number can be found in *The Hospital and Health Services Year Book* which is updated annually and will be in the public library.

The following lists some centres in the United Kingdom where there are Breast Units and Clinics, staffed by medical personnel who specialize in diseases of the breast:

Bath – Royal United Hospital
Birmingham – Selly Oak Hospital
Bradford – Royal Infirmary
Guildford – Royal Surrey County Hospital
Hartlepool – General Hospital
Huddersfield – St Luke's Hospital
Leeds – General Infirmary
Liverpool – General Infirmary
Manchester – Withington Hospital and Christie
Newcastle – General Hospital
Nottingham – General Hospital
Oxford – Radcliffe Infirmary
Southampton – Southampton Hospital
West Sussex – King Edward VII Hospital, Midhurst

Northern Ireland
Belfast – Royal Victoria Hospital

Scotland
Dundee – Ninewells Hospital
Edinburgh – The Royal Infirmary
Glasgow – Gartnavel, Western Infirmary

Wales
Cardiff – University Hospital of Wales

London
Charing Cross Hospital, SW6
Guy's Hospital, SE1
Hammersmith Hospital, W12
King's College Hospital, SE5
Middlesex Hospital, Radiotherapy Institute, W1
Royal Free Hospital, NW3
Royal Marsden, SW6, and Sutton, Surrey
St Mary's Hospital, W2
St Thomas's Hospital, SE1
University College Hospital, WC1
Private Clinics offering complete screening service

BUPA
Battlebridge House
300 Grays Inn Road
London WC1
01-837 6484

BUPA Medical Centre
Warwick House
17-19 Warwick Road
Old Trafford
Manchester M16 0QQ
061-872 7717/8

Both these centres offer a special Health Screening Service for women which comprises a breast and pelvic check. Thermography is done automatically and mammography if it is considered necessary. Two more centres are being opened in Spring 1982:

BUPA Medical Centre
Stafford Lodge
Chesterfield Hospital
Clifton Hill
Bristol
0272 731 433

BUPA Medical Centre
29 Smallbrook Queensway
Birmingham
021 632 6738

The Cavendish Medical Centre Ltd
99 New Cavendish Street
London W1M 7FQ
01-637 8941 (10 lines)

Offers a similar special service for women called Womanscreen.

Women's Cancer Detection Society
Queen Elizabeth Hospital
Gateshead
Tyne and Wear

This society runs a private clinic at the above hospital which is charitably financed and offers a full screening service for breast cancer at a nominal fee. Available only to women living in the North of England.

Other useful addresses

Women's National Cancer Control Campaign
1 South Audley Street
London W1Y 5DQ
01-499 7532/4

Promotes measures for the early detection of cancer of the cervix and of the breast through health education and a free screening service by means of a fleet of mobile clinics. (Manual examination only of the breast.) Distributes free illustrated leaflets on breast self-examination and has also made a film on the same subject called 'Your Life in Your Hands'. If you would like to offer your services for fund-raising or require information, including the address of your nearest Local Authority Clinic, contact the Information Officer at the above address.

The Mastectomy Association
1 Colworth Road
Croydon CR0 7AD
01-654 8643

Self-help group of volunteers, all post-mastectomy patients, who will give practical advice and information to women who have recently had a mastectomy.

Cancer Information Association
Marygold House
Carfax
Oxford OX1 1EF
Oxford 46654

Health Education service. Runs lectures and conferences.

Also:
C.A.R.E. (Cancer Patient Aftercare)
Lodge Cottage
Church Lane
Timsbury
Bath BA3 1LF

Patientcare Mastectomy Centres

Offer a private fitting and consultative service to women who have had a mastectomy. Has a wide range of breast forms (prostheses) some of which are not available through the National Health Service and also has special lines in swimwear and night-wear. Offices with trained fitter at the following addresses:

Room 213
Bond Street House
14 Clifford Street
London W1X 1RE
01-491 4118

15/16 George IV Bridge
Edinburgh EH1 1EL.
031-226 5125

121 Douglas Street
Glasgow G2 4HE
041-332 4414

22 Union Street
Dundee DD1 4BH
0382 21593

8/10 Union Street
Inverness IV1 1PL
0463 36691

Marie Curie Memorial Foundation
124 Sloane Street
London SW1
01-730 9157

Funds research. Runs educational and welfare programmes
including nursing homes for cancer patients.

National Society for Cancer Relief
Michael Sobell House
30 Dorset Square
London NW1
01-402 8125

Provides practical help to cancer patients and their families.

Regional Cancer Services in Leeds, Manchester, South West
Thames and Wessex offer advice and information. Contact your
local Area Health Authority for addresses.

Cancer Research Organizations
Cancer Research Campaign
2 Carlton House Terrace
London SW17 5AR
01-930 8972

Faith Courtauld Unit for Human Studies in Cancer
King's College Hospital
Denmark Hill
London SE5

Imperial Cancer Research Fund
Lincoln's Inn Fields
London WC2
01-242 0200

Tenovus
111 Cathedral Road
Cardiff
Wales
Cardiff 42851 (Information)

Bibliography

The reader will find most of the source material for this book in the general bibliography which I have divided into two categories – *lay* and *medical*. Where I have referred to specific medical papers discussing a particular aspect of treatment or research, I have listed them under the appropriate chapter.

General

1 Lay

The Invisible Worm by Rosamund Campion (Macmillan, New York, 1972).

What Women Should Know About the Breast Cancer Controversy by George Crile Jr MD (Pocket Books, New York).

What We Know About Cancer by R. J. C. Harris (George Allen & Unwin, 1970).

Breast Cancer: A Personal History and an Investigative Report by Rose Kushner (Harcourt Brace Jovanovich, New York, 1975).

Reach to Recovery by Terese Lasser and William Kendall Clarke (Simon & Schuster, 1972).

Rehabilitation of Mastectomy Patients by June Marchant (William Heinemann Medical Books, 1978).

Three Weeks in Spring by Joan H. Parker and Robert B. Parker (André Deutsch, 1978).

Mastectomy, A Patient's Guide to Coping with Breast Surgery by Nancy Robinson and Ian Swash (Thorson's Publishers Ltd, 1977).

First, You Cry by Betty Rollin (Signet, New York, 1977).

Illness as Metaphor by Susan Sontag (McGraw-Hill Ryerson Ltd, Canada, and Farrar, Straus and Giroux, New York, 1978).

But Why Cancer, Sally? by Dr Basil Stoll (William Heinemann Medical Books, 1976).

The Female Breast by Elizabeth Weiss (Bantam Books, New York, 1975).

2 *Medical*
Stress, Psychological Factors and Cancer, an annotated collection of readings from the professional literature with bibliography. Compiled and edited by Jeanne Acheerberg, PhD, Carl Simonton MD and Stephanie Matthews-Simonton (New Medicine Press, Texas, 1976).

A Nutritional Approach to Cancer. Proceedings of a conference organized by the East West Foundation at Pine Manor College, Chestnut Hill, Massachusetts, 9 March 1977.

The Treatment of Breast Cancer, edited by Prof. Sir Hedley Atkins, KBE (Medical and Technical Publishing, 1974).

Understanding Cancer, a guide for the Caring Professions by Ian Burn and Roger L. Meyrick (HMSO, 1977).

Cancer, the Behavioural Dimensions, edited by Joseph W. Cullen, Bernard H. Fox and Ruby N. Isom (Raven Press, New York).

Mammography, Thermography and Ultrasonography in Breast Disease by K. T. Evans and I. H. Gravelle (Butterworths, 1973).

Diseases of the Breast by C. D. Haagensen, MD, revised edition (W. B. Saunders, 1971).

Report of the Joint Working Group on Oral Contraceptives (HMSO, 1976).

Diagnosis and Treatment of Breast Lesions by Henry P. Leis Jr MD (H. K. Lewis and Co, 1970).

Seeds of Destruction. The Scientific Report on Cancer Research by Thomas H. Maugh and Jean L. Marx (Plenum Press, New York, 1975).

Breast Cancer: Advances in Research and Treatment, Vol I: Current Approaches to Therapy, edited by William L. McGuire MD (Churchill Livingstone, 1977).

Breast Cancer. Edited from the Proceedings of the International Breast Cancer Conference held in Lucerne, Switzerland 31 July to 4 August 1976, by Montague, Stonesifer and Lewison (Alan R. Liss, Inc, New York, 1977).

Host Defences in Breast Cancer, edited by Basil A. Stoll (William Heinemann Medical Books, 1975).

Breast Cancer Management, Early and Late, edited by Basil A. Stoll (William Heinemann Medical Books, 1977).

Secondary Spread in Breast Cancer, edited by Basil A. Stoll (William Heinemann Medical Books, 1977).

Steroid Contraception and the Risk of Neoplasia. Report of WHO Scientific Group, Technical Report Series 619 (WHO, Geneva, 1978).

Chapter references

1 Bosom thoughts
Modesty in Dress: an Inquiry into the Fundamentals of Fashion by James Laver (William Heinemann, 1969).

2 A royal curse
'Psychological Attributes of Women Who Develop Breast Cancer; a controlled study' by S. Greer and Tina Morris, *Journal of Psychosomatic Research*, Vol 19 (November 1974), pp 147–53.

'Breast Cancer and Reproductive History of Women in South Wales' by C. R. Lowe and Brian MacMahon, *Lancet* (24 January 1970), pp 153–7.

'A *Type C* for Cancer?' by Tina Morris. Paper delivered at The Royal Society of Medicine, Clinical Oncology Study Course, London, September 1977.

'Female Hormones and Cancer of the Breast' by Martin Vessey. Paper in *Epidemiological Evaluation of Drugs*, edited by F. Colombo et al (Elsevier/North Holland Biomedical Press, Amsterdam).

3 What are we looking for?
'Applied Research in Teaching Breast Self-Examination' by Patricia Hobbs, *Health Education Journal 2*, Vol 32 (1973).

4 I've got a lump in my breast
'Radiological Investigation of Breast Disease' by I. H. Gravelle, *British Medicine* (1977).

'How to Help the 1 in 4 with Breast Lumps Who Delay Presenting' by S. Greer, *Modern Medicine* (April 1978).

'Psychological Aspects: Delay in the Treatment of Breast Cancer' by
S. Greer, *Proceedings of the Royal Society of Medicine*, Vol 67, No 6
(June 1974), pp 470–73.

'Breast Cancer: How a GP Can Aid Early Detection' by Henry P. Leis,
Modern Medicine (March 1978).

'How Mammography Can Aid Your Diagnosis' by J. L. Price,
Modern Medicine (March 1978).

5 To screen or not to screen?
'Breast Cancer': Contribution to *Screening in Medical Care* by
C. R. Lowe (Oxford University Press, 1968).

'Cancer Screening in Reducing Mortality from Breast Cancer' by
Sam Shapiro, Philip Strax MD and Louis Venet MD, *The Journal of
the American Medical Association*, Vol 215, No 11 (15 March 1971).

'Practical Mass Screening for Early Breast Cancer ' by Philip Strax
MD (Guttman Institute, New York, 1972).

'Screening for Breast Cancer'. Report from Edinburgh Breast
Screening Clinic, *British Medical Journal* (15 July 1978).

'Screening for Breast Cancer'. Statement by British Breast Group,
British Medical Journal (15 July 1978). See also leading article in same
issue.

8 Is your operation really necessary?
'Simple Mastectomy and Pectoral Node Biopsy' by Forrest, Roberts,
Cant and Shiva, *British Journal of Surgery*, Vol 63, No 8 (August
1976), pp 569–75.

NB The clinical staging classification for breast cancer is based on the
criteria established by the American Joint Committee for Cancer
Staging and End Results Reporting, September 1973.

9 A new hope
'Reconstruction of the Breast as a Primary and Secondary Procedure
following Mastectomy for Carcinoma' by G. T. Watts, *British
Journal of Surgery*, Vol 63, No 10 (October 1976), pp 823–6.

'Restorative Prosthetic Mammaplasty in Mastectomy for Carcinoma
and Benign Lesions' by G. T. Watts, *Clinics in Plastic Surgery*, Vol 3,
No 2 (April 1976).

10 What else can they do?
'Combination Chemotherapy as an Adjuvant Treatment in Operable Breast Cancer' by Gianni Bonadonna et al, *New England Journal of Medicine*, Vol 294, No 8 (19 February 1976).

11 Informed consent
'Design and Analysis of Randomized Clinical Trials Requiring Prolonged Observation of Each Patient' by R. Peto, M. C. Pike et al, 'Part I – Introduction and Design', *British Journal of Cancer* (1976), 34.585, and 'Part II – Analysis and Examples', *British Journal of Cancer* (1977), 35.1.

12 Your mind
'Treatment of Breast Cancer: Doctor Patient Communication and Psycho-Social Implications' by Edward S. Chesser and John L. Anderson. Paper presented to the Psychiatry Section of the Royal Society of Medicine, 11 February 1975.

'The Psychological and Social Sequelae of Mastectomy' by Peter Maguire. A chapter in *Modern Perspectives in the Psychiatric Aspects of Surgery* edited by John G. Howells (Brunner/Mazel Inc, New York, 1976).

'Psychiatric Problems in the First Year after Mastectomy' by Peter Maguire, E. G. Lee et al, *British Medical Journal* (15 April 1978).

'Psychological and Social Adjustment to Mastectomy – a two-year follow-up study ' by Tina Morris, S. Greer et al, *Cancer*, Vol 40, No 5 (November 1977).

The Effect of Psychosocial Milieu in the Treatment of Cancer by M. L. S. Vachon, A. Formo et al (Paper presented at Columbia University, New York City, February 1977).

'Applying Psychiatric Techniques to Patients with Cancer' by M. L. S Vachon and W. A. Lyall, *Hospital and Community Psychiatry*, Vol 27, No 8, pp 582–4, 1976.

The Use of Group Meetings with Cancer Patients and Their Families by M. L. S. Vachon and W. A. Lyall et al, in *Cancer, Stress and Death* (Plenum Press, New York, 1979).

Index